MW00513821

A Natural History of Birds. Most of Which Have not Been Figur'd or Describ'd, and Others Very Little Known ... Containing the Figures of Sixty Birds and two Quadrupedes, Engrav'd on Fifty-two Copper Plates, Exactly Colour'd of 4

The
the Revd Dr Birch
Present

from his Obliged
Humble Servant —
— the Author

April 26 1758

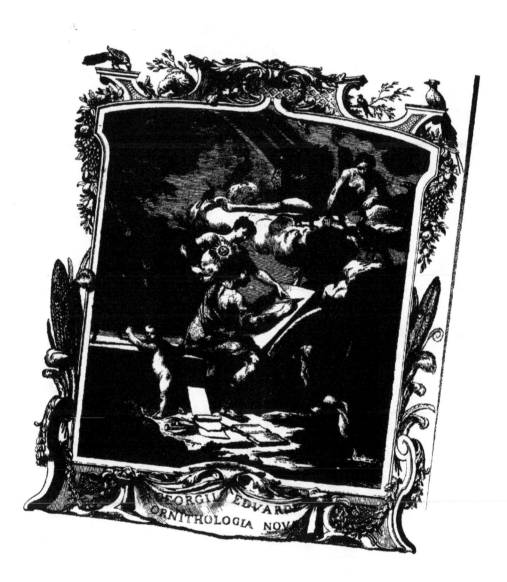

GEORGII EDVARDI
ORNITHOLOGIA NOV

A

NATURAL HISTORY

OF

B I R D S.

Moſt of which have not been figur'd or deſcrib'd, and others very little known from obſcure or too brief Deſcriptions without Figures, or from Figures very ill deſign'd.

CONTAINING

The Figures of Sixty BIRDS and Two QUADRUPEDES, engrav'd on Fifty-two Copper Plates, after curious Original Drawings from Life, and exactly Colour'd. With full and accurate Deſcriptions.

By GEORGE EDWARDS.

Natura. ſemper eadem, ſed Artes ſunt variæ.

L O N D O N:

Printed for the AUTHOR, at the *College of Phyſicians* in *Warwick-Lane.*
M.DCC.XLIII.

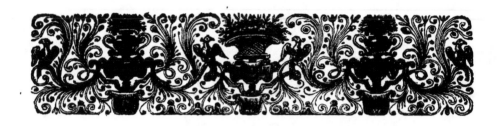

To the Honourable the

PRESIDENT and FELLOWS

OF THE

Royal College of PHYSICIANS, *of* LONDON.

Honoured SIRS,

HE juſt Senſe I have of Your great Learning and profound Judgment in all the Sciences, and my own Ignorance in moſt of them, might deter me from Preſenting this Trifle, was I not encouraged by Your great Goodneſs and Willingneſs to cheriſh and give Life to the leaſt Spark of Knowledge You perceive kindling in any one, tho' of inferior Rank ; which Benevolence in You removes that Fear, that otherwiſe would forbid my Approach. This Work hath, indeed, receiv'd its very Being from your Smiles ; for the favourable Reception my firſt Eſſays in this Way, ſome-time ago preſented to the College met with, hath

A 2 encouraged

encouraged me to publish this History of BIRDS, which would otherwise have continued in Obscurity; so that I may esteem Your Honours, in some measure, Parents of it; therefore I humbly beg You would please to favour it with your Patronage, which I shall always esteem its greatest Merit.   I shall forbear to enter upon the Excellencies and Virtues of your Honourable Society, since the World is, by Experience, thoroughly convinced of Your publick Usefulness and Worth.

But it would be inexcusable in me, should I slip this Opportunity, publickly to acknowledge the many and great Favours I have received from Your Hands, as a Publick Body, such as generous Gratuities for slight Services, and many other Privileges and Conveniencies, over and above the Salary of my Office : I have not only received these publick Kindnesses, but innumerable private Favours from the illustrious Members of Your honourable Society, who have furnish'd me with all Things necessary to forward me in this Work, and have freely given me their Advice and Instructions.   For these many and great Favours, I cannot conclude without acknowledging, with a grateful Mind, the many Obligations You have laid upon him who is in a particular Manner,

HONOURED SIRS,

Your most Dutiful,

and most obliged humble Servant,

GEORGE EDWARDS.

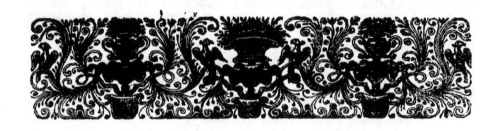

THE

PREFACE.

THE *Wisdom and Power of God are manifest to all Rational Creatures, from a Contemplation of his wonderful Works in the Creation of this World: He hath formed every Beast of the Field, Bird of the Air, and Fish of the Waters: He hath also formed every Tree and Plant; every creeping Insect was made by Him. All that the Earth, Air, or Waters produce were created by God's Power. Now Man being the only rational Being in this World, it seemeth plain by natural Light, that the Dominion of all Creatures was given to him by God; therefore since Man's Obligation to God is greater than that of any other Creature, his Acts of Humiliation, Adoration and Gratitude ought to be in some degree proportionable to the Favour and Benefits he hath received. Amongst the many Acts of Gratitude we owe to God, it may be accounted one, to study and contemplate the Perfections and Beauties of his Works of Creation. Every new Discovery must necessarily raise in us a fresh Sense of the Greatness, Wisdom and Power of God: He hath so order'd Things that almost every Part of*

[*a*] *the*

the Creation is for our Benefit, either to the Support of our Being, the Delight of our Senses, or the agreeable Exercise of the rational Faculty. If there are some few poisonous Animals and Plants fatal to Man, these may serve to heighten the contrary Blessings; since we could have no Idea of Benefits, were we insensible of their Contraries; and seeing God has given us Reason by which we are able to choose the Good and avoid the Evil, we suffer very little from the malignant Parts of the Creation.

God hath given to brutal Animals a certain Law whereby to govern themselves, which is called an Instinct, it being an inward implanted Tendency to particular Actions, from which they cannot stray. This Instinct or inward Force appears to be stronger in Brutes than in the human Species, and supplies to them the defect of Reason. Man hath an Instinct also, but much weaker than that in other Animals, but to make up that Want God hath given him a glimmering of that heavenly Light, called Reason. Now as Man was design'd Lord of this lower World, and the Possession of every Part thereof was given to him, the Instinct of Brutes would not have been sufficient, nor would Reason itself have been enough without some inward Appetites; for without Instinct his Generation would probably have soon been at an end; and we should have neglected the Support of our individual Bodies, had we only Reason, and not Hunger to tell us, that Eating was necessary to Life.

Reason is our director, when we change our Country from one extreme Climate to another: The Russian tho' inclosed in close Houses firmly secur'd against the penetration of the cold Air, and inwardly heated with Stoves, when he travels into Persia and India, is directed by the same Reason to sleep in the open Air, and on the Tops of Houses, and to use Machines to agitate and bring fresh Air about him; and on the contrary the Ethiopian, tho' his Lodging be in the open Plains and Deserts, and he without any Clothing, yet when he is brought to Europe, he is glad to screen himself in warm Houses, and warm himself by Fires, and cover himself with thick Clothing. Reason giveth Man this Pre-eminence over brute Beasts; by it he can make almost all Parts of the World habitable to him by Arts and Inventions to screen himself from the great Heats in some Parts, and defend himself from the piercing Colds in other Parts of the World. No brute Animal can thus indifferently inhabit any Part of

the

the World, because their innate Laws are unchangeable, and accommodated only to such Climates as Nature has placed them in; so that I believe there is no Creature whose Race is spread in all habitable Parts of the World, as is that of the human Species. Each Animal seems to have his appointed Climate, out of which, if he be removed to one far different, his Generation ceaseth or loseth its first Properties, whereas such Creatures as continue where Nature placed them, vary hardly at all from the Species from which they sprang, preserving the same Magnitude, Form and Colours throughout all Ages; for it seemeth as if God had set particular marks of Distinction on each Species from which they cannot stray.

From this Reason I found the agreement between each different Generation of Animal and Plant, which always continues to bear the Form and Likeness of those in which they were first inclosed. Indeed some domestick Animals and Plants differ in some sort from their first Parents, which were savage. I take these Differences not to be very material, and to proceed from the unnatural Food, Habitation, and other Circumstances that may alter the Plant or Animal in Magnitude or Colour; which is not material; seeing these Things so made domestick, if turned again to their native Habitations in a Generation or two cast off those Accidents attain'd by unnatural Situations, and recover their first Forms and Colours stamped on them in the first Creation of the whole Species.

Many who have wrote in former Times on Nature, suppose that all Things which were at first created by God on this Globe, have been ever since, by his Providence, continued through an implanted seminal Power down to these Times, and will continue as long as the Earth endureth; yet some great Naturalists in these Days are quite of a different Opinion, and their Reasons for these Opinions are founded on the great Variety of fossil Substances found daily in many Parts of the World, resembling Animals and Parts of Animals now in being, as well as Animals and Parts of Animals not to be met with by the most laborious Searches of the Curious.

From the general face of Things we may safely conclude there have been great Revolutions on the Face of this Earth, which in many Places seem to have been caused by a great Quantity of Water prevailing, and passing very swiftly over its Surface, breaking up its lower Parts, and

tearing

rearing them into Mountains, and carrying other Parts which have lain high into the Sea; so that in many Places we find buried in high Mountains far Inland, Substances which received their first Formation in the Sea, and in some low Grounds deep buried near the Sea, we find many Things that received their first Forms in the Mountains. It is probable some of these great Revolutions might be so wide spread at once, as utterly to extinguish some Animals that were in God's original Creation of this World.

If we consider the beautiful Parts of Nature, so far as they charm the Sight by the lustre and variety of Colours, and the fineness of the Texture of Parts, I think many will agree, that the fine Things produced may charm the Eye, as much as the most studied and harmonious Compositions in Musick can charm the Ear. But it is common to say, that People who have no delight in Musick, have no Ear: And I think, we may as justly say of those who are no ways moved to Admiration, when the Beauties of Nature present themselves, that they want Eyes. Whether or not Nature design'd the beautiful Forms and Colourings we perceive in several kinds of Insects and other Animals, as things to delight and please the Sense of those Animals and others of the brute Creation: Or whether they were design'd principally for the Delight and Contemplation of Man the Lord of this lower World, is a Question. A Reason in my Opinion, why Insects are not sensible of their own Beauty, is the Form of their Eyes, which let in the Light through a kind of Net-work, which must discover the Objects in a confused manner; or if we suppose each little part a distinct Eye, they are so small that an Object must almost touch them, to be distinctly perceived in its Parts, and the Quantity taken in at once so small, that the intire Form of one Insect can hardly appear plain to another; these Eyes may indeed serve them to distinguish opake Bodies from the clear Air they fly in, and when they approach very near to pick out small Particles lying on Leaves and Fruits which supply most Insects with Food.

Now seeing the Eyes of Man seem to be more adapted than those of Insects to receive the various Forms and Colours of natural Things, I am of Opinion that God principally design'd these things not only to please and delight the outward Senses of Man, but that the Contemplation of them

should

should point out to the Mind the surprising Manner of God's Method of working who created all things; and this may serve as natural Arguments of his infinite Wisdom and Power.

Mr. Horsley *in his* Britannia Romana, *making a sort of Apology for that Work in his Preface, has these Words, which will not be amiss to quote for my present Purpose.* " I have always looked on it as an In-
" stance of divine Wisdom, that it should be so order'd that different
" Men have such different Tastes and Inclinations. By this means the
" several Parts of Knowledge are more cultivated: And I think we owe
" our Thanks to any one, who will apply himself to the Study of any
" particular Thing; though it seem minute, and may not suit our
" Taste or Inclination to pursue it ourselves. This gives us, at least,
" an Opportunity of knowing on easier Terms what can be said on that
" Subject."

It is always necessary that every Age should labour to discover something, and not sit down content with the Discoveries of our Forefathers, for Experience shews the Knowledge of our Ancestors dwindles away, and decays daily; for such is the nature of Time, that it obscures or destroys the Knowledge of past Ages by the many wasteful Events which happen in a long course of Years, such as Fire, Rapine, Inundations, Loss of the Liberties of Countries, and many other Things. But more than all these, the change of Languages affects our Knowledge; for no Language continues the same for many Centuries: Inscriptions indeed have continued some Thousands of Years, but when the Languages are dead in which they are wrote, the Sense of them by Ages becomes darker and darker, till at last they are utterly obscure, as we find the most antient are, witness the Monuments of the antient Egyptians, *the Ruins of* Persepolis, *and other mighty Ruins in many Parts of the World: So that we see we cannot depend on the Knowledge of the Antients as a perpetual Fund; we must, as Times go, gather what we can from them, and add to it as much as we can of our own, that we may keep up the Stock we have by adding something in the room of what must inevitably be lost; for if we sit down content with what is already known, which is a Knowledge we are sure is decreasing every Day, we in a few Ages may know nothing, and be reduced to a state equal to the wild* Americans, *since we know that* Europe

itself

itself hath been well nigh reduced to such a State a few Centuries ago by falling into a superstitious Lethargy, neglecting all farther Improvements of Knowledge, and despising Reason, Nature and the evidence of Sense.

Every one ought to attain to as high a degree of natural Knowledge as he can, for a deep Knowledge in Nature has detected many false Pretenders to Inspiration, Prophesy, and the like, while the Ignorant in Nature and her Laws have been deluded by the meanest and lowest Pretenders, such as diabolical Possessions, fantastical Apparitions, Dreams, good and bad, Omens, and the like.

As Arts have been brought by gradual Steps from one degree of Perfection to another, by joining the Knowledge of past Times left us in the Writings of those that are gone before, with the Discoveries and Experience of the present Times; so even the knowledge of Nature itself hath been multiply'd by the various degrees of Conception, and different Powers of Penetration that have been given by God through past Ages to Mankind, which have been handed down through the Records of Time to us. Without this Knowledge of other Men joined to our own, our Knowledge would be like that of savage People who live together in small Tribes or Families, and have nothing but meer mother Wit and pure natural Capacity, chiefly derived from the Senses, to direct them, they not knowing what any of their Ancestors said or thought before them for want of Characters to express Words; so that each Man's Knowledge is his own, or has little assistance from others: I do not mean that while we are searching into Nature's Works, we should neglect the curious Arts and Inventions of Men; for by being well skill'd in Arts we are enabled the better to make Discoveries in Nature. Besides, a fine Art lost may never be recover'd, but Nature, tho' at present unknown by searching, may at one time or other be found, because she always endureth and continueth the same. Art and Nature, like two Sisters, should always walk hand in hand, that so they may reciprocally aid and assist each other.

He who goes into foreign Parts, in order to improve himself in natural Knowledge or other Sciences, should first acquire all that may be learned in his own Country, lest he should expose himself, as many have done, by going abroad, telling us at their return many such things as were already

known,

known, or might have been easily discovered in our own Country. To produce an Instance of this, let any one knowing in Birds turn over Cornelius le Bruyn's *Travels into* Muscovy, Persia, &c. *there he will find described the* Spoon-bill, *call'd in the* Russian *Language* Calpetse, *Vol.* 1. *P.* 91. *of the* English *Translation. The* Bald Coot, *call'd in the* Persian, Paes-jelek, *Vol.* 1. *P.* 182. *The* Pelican, *call'd by the* Russians, Babbe *or* Water-Carrier, *Vol.* 2. *P.* 167. *Now these Birds being all very well described by natural Historians, they need no farther Descriptions; but he did not mean to give us things before described, but, through Ignorance in that particular Part of natural History, supposed these Birds altogether unknown, since he has not given them their common* European *Names; it is surprizing he should not know the* Spoon-bill, *because those who have described it make it a Native of* Holland, *and tell the Place where it builds and breeds. It is still more strange he should go to* Ispahan *to figure and describe the* Bald Coot, *which abounds in every Canal and Dike round about the* Hague *the Place of his Birth: It shews a fond Inclination to discover the Rarities of foreign Countries, before a Person has attained the Knowledge of what is to be known in his native Country: which is to begin where one should end; so that all People who go abroad on any Discoveries should be qualified as abovementioned, but more particularly all should inform themselves, as far as may be, at home, in those things they expresly go to make farther Discoveries of. For want of such Qualifications, and through dishonest Principles, Vice and Indolence, many who have been sent abroad at the Expence of others, have in no sort answered the Expectations of those who sent them, which hath discouraged Gentlemen of Curiosity and Fortune from advancing Money on such fruitless Expeditions.*

Nevertheless some Men thus sent, have with great labour and honesty answer'd the Expectations of their Patrons. It would be very proper for all Travellers into foreign Parts, to take notice of what Birds and Beasts they find, and at what Seasons of the Year they find them, and at what Times they disappear, and when they appear again, that so we may in time give a tolerable account of the Places to which Birds and Beasts of Passage go that are found with us, and in other Countries only at certain Seasons of the Year. Many may think perhaps that there are no Beasts of Passage, but I have been informed by a Person of Reputation, who now resides in one of the English *Forts in* Hudson's-Bay, *that the Deer in that Country pass northward in the beginning of Summer, and return to the South at the approach of Winter, and that they pass in certain beaten Tracts well known to the Indians, as well as the* English *residing there, who lie in wait for them, and kill great Numbers for their Skins. They are said by the Natives to pass very far North in the Summer, and to return in the Winter far enough Southward to come to a temperate Climate. I have in my Searches after Birds discover'd some few that are found in* England *at certain Seasons, to be found also in* Bengal; *and some found in* Europe, *tho' not in* England, *are found also in* Bengal: *Whether they continue there all the Year, or are only Birds of Passage, as they are with us, I cannot tell; but it would be worth the Observation of any curious* Englishman *residing in that Country; therefore I shall set down their Names, viz.*

The Greater Redstart,	Merula Saxatilis, *Aldrov.*
The Witwal,	Icterus, *Plinii,*
The Wheat-Ear,	Oenanthe *or* Vitiflora,
The Small-Green-Wren,	Regulus non cristatus,
The House-Swallow,	Hirundo domestica,
The Bee-eater,	Merops,
The Wry-neck,	Iynx *or* Torquilla.

Of this Number the Wheat-Ear, *the* Green Wren, *the* House-Swallow *and* Wry-neck, *are found in* England *in Summer, and all of them in the Southern Parts of* Europe, *where I believe they are Birds of Passage also. All these I have met with in Parcels of Birds sent from* Bengal; *and if any Person of good Observation in* India *could discover that these Birds are absent there while present with us, and present there whilst absent here, it would answer the Question, whither and in what manner do these Birds pass?*

It is indeed my Opinion, that all those Birds which are seen with us only some part of the Year, pass into other Countries when they are out of our sight. We are certain some of them must, because they do not breed while they continue with us; these are the Wood-cock, Snipes, Field-fare, Redwing *and some others: These I believe, go into northern Countries*

*to breed. The Summer Birds of Paſſage alſo come from more ſouthern
Countries northward to us, and breed here: Seeing then Birds retire from
more northern Parts to winter with us, why ſhould not tender Birds who
viſit us in Summer and breed here, retire and ſhelter themſelves in
ſouthern Countries, where they are ſecure from cold, which they cannot
bear, and find ſuch Food as is natural to them. But many would make
Sleepers of them, and ſay they retire to holes under Ground, and in
hollow Trees, &c. and that they are ſo fat that they cannot fly far at
the Times they diſappear, which Fatneſs I take rather for a providential
Proviſion, to enable them to take a flight of many Days without being
quite exhauſted and ſpent. A farther Reaſon to me, that our Summer
Birds who diſappear are not Sleepers, is, that no ſuch ſleeping Birds
have at any time been found, and all the reports of theſe things are ſo
uncertain, that no ſober Man can at all depend on them: Did they
really creep into holes as is reported, it would be certainly known, and
not remain, as it does, a very doubtful Matter; for why ſhould they not
be daily found ſleeping, as are Dormice, by Wood-men and Country
People, ſince many of the ſuppoſed Sleepers are found awake in much
greater Numbers. I believe indeed that the Inſtinct of theſe Birds is
not ſo abſolutely certain, as to prevent them from being ſometimes ſur-
priſed by a very cold wet Autumn: In ſuch a caſe I believe ſome Flocks
of* Swallows *have loſt their Paſſage, and have been conſtrain'd through
Weakneſs to ſhelter themſelves in holes where they have periſhed.*

*Natural Hiſtory cannot in any degree be perfect without Figures;
therefore I think we ſhould promote Drawing, in all ſuch young People
who ſeem to have a liking to it; no one need think it an Amuſement
beneath his Dignity, ſince our preſent Royal Family and many of the
young Nobility have been inſtructed in that Art. The World may
perhaps think I ſay this in order to promote my ſelf; becauſe hitherto I
have taught young Gentlemen and Ladies to draw; but to take away
ſuch Imputation, I purpoſe to decline any thing of that ſort which may
hereafter offer. Every one who conſults antient Authors, is very ſenſible
of their Deficiencies in the want of Figures; for many things are mention'd by a bare Name without any Deſcription or Figure, and great
phyſical Virtues and other Uſes are attributed to ſome of theſe things,*

[c] *but*

but there being no certain Marks to shew what things in Nature were called by those Names, we have now wholly lost them, or take different things for them, or are in dispute about them; therefore Authors, Naturalists especially, should consult, first of all, the outward Forms of things in order farther to explain them by Descriptions and other Marks; and deliver them down to Posterity, so as to free them, so far as human Reason is capable of, from the Losses and Injuries they may sustain from Time. In describing natural Things nothing ought to be omitted, that is any way remarkable, and may fix and establish the Character of the thing described, so as plainly to distinguish it from all other things: This may be done without following the minute Steps of some Authors, who have wrote large Books on single Birds or Plants, for long Descriptions lead the Mind into Mazes and Confusion, and tire rather than instruct. On the other hand too brief Descriptions should be avoided; for very often these are found to consist only of such general Forms and Colourings that are common to many things of the same Genus, with the thing so briefly described, which makes the Description uncertain, or rather no natural Description at all. If Naturalists would observe this medium, and study a plain comprehensive Language, and well expressing the Things treated of, they might gradually, by making the Study both useful and pleasant, bring many into the love of Natural History, who now despise it.

I know there are some Gentlemen, that put the Terms of mean and little upon such Sciences or Studies that they themselves have no Taste for; and others would make them useless by calling them mere Speculations. Natural History has been particularly aspersed and treated in this manner by the Enemies to all Knowledge, but such as brings with it immediate Profit or sensual Pleasure: But if these Gentlemen will look back a little, they will find that Men as great, as wise and magnanimous, at least as themselves, in all Ages, have busied themselves in the Discoveries and Knowledge of Nature. King Soloman is a great Example in this matter, who was himself a natural Historian, and perhaps had penetrated farther into Nature than any one has done since. Alexander the Great was remarkable for encouraging all the fine Arts, as well natural History as other Literature, without which his Memory could not have subsisted till this Time. But to come nearer our own Times,

Lewis

Lewis XIV. *of* France, *tho' one of the greatest Princes of the Age he lived in, and engaged in several Wars for a considerable Part of his Life, yet found time to improve his Mind by the Study of the fine Arts, and established an Academy for the farther Improvement of Arts and new Discoveries in Nature:* He was such a Lover of the Productions of Nature, that he made Gardens and built magnificent Stoves, &c. for the raising and reception of all Exotick Plants, and built at Versailles near his Palace, an elegant and curious Place called the Managery, with large Apartments and Conveniencies for the Reception of living Animals from all Parts of the World, and not only rare Pictures and Sculptures of the greatest Masters were collected in his Cabinets, but several extraordinary Productions of Nature. Augustus *the late King of* Poland was also a great Encourager of natural Knowledge, and had gather'd a large Collection of natural Productions from most Parts of the World.

They who draw after Nature, on account of Natural History, should represent things justly and according to Nature, and not strive to exalt or raise her above herself; for by so doing, instead of instructing, they will lead the World into Errors; nor can the Works of two Authors on the same Subject ever agree. The historical Painter, especially he that would represent the Fictions of the Poets, may take greater Liberties, and study by all Methods to elevate his Subject by adding the highest Strokes of Art, in order to please the Eye, and raise in the Mind Ideas equal to the Historian or Poet he would represent: Yet every one who reads Natural History, and sees Figures and Descriptions of things in Nature, supposes they are, or ought to have been immediately drawn and described from Nature. But no experienced Man, when he beholds an historical Piece, supposes the Figures there drawn, are like to those they are intended to represent either in Feature or Person, any farther than in general the Historian or Poet may have told us, that one Man was a graceful Person, another a little crooked or deformed, which Accidents a Painter has liberty to carry to what degree of Perfection or Imperfection he can conceive, provided alway he doth not contradict the Letter of his Historian. But in drawing after Nature a most religious and scrupulous Strictness is to be observed, and by this means only we can demonstrate, that Nature is or is not the same through all Times. If Natural

Historians,

Historians, or they who draw for them, would carefully observe these Rules, some of them might perhaps produce Figures that would be deemed perfect by the knowing Naturalists of these Times, and escape their Censure; then might they, like the celebrated Statues of the antient Greeks and Romans, pass down as Models to future Ages, as things justly and truly representing Nature; but these things are rather to be wished for than expected.

It is time to say something, by way of Apology, for the following Descriptions of Birds I have been collecting for more than Twenty Years, and have been for a good part of the Time employ'd by many curious Gentlemen in London *to draw such rare foreign Birds as they were possess'd of, and never neglected to take Draughts of them with their Permission, for my own Collection; and having stored up some hundreds, I shewed them from time to time to curious Gentlemen who favour'd me with their Visits, and in looking them over several of them have told me, that there were many amongst them that had not been figured or described by any Author, and that it would be worth my while to publish them; but I was backward in resolving to do it, because I knew not so much of many of the Birds, as to know from what Country they came, which is very material in Natural History. They answer'd, that as I had taken the Draughts from Nature, and that it could be well attested, and the like Birds might perhaps never be met with again, it was better to preserve the Figures without knowing their Countries than not at all. I have not had the Advantage of being in the Countries out of* Europe *where any of the Birds I have described are found, as some present Writers of Natural History have; but I have taken all the pains in my Power to make my Descriptions as perfect as the nature of the thing will admit of. I have been particularly careful never to speak in the Affirmative, but where I was fully satisfied I was in the right. The far greater part of these Descriptions are from Birds never before described: There are indeed some few which have been described, but not figured, and some that have been very ill figured and described before; but I have not drawn or described any thing that was done before in any tolerable degree of Perfection; so that these Draughts and Descriptions may be looked on as new. I have not transcribed the Descriptions out of other Authors*

without

without acknowledging from whence I had them, as a late Publisher of a great Number of coloured Birds has done; but always chose to have old Descriptions farthest from my Mind, when I described any thing, because I thought Nature herself the best Director. I have indeed, as I ought, consulted Men and Books, in order to gain all the Light I could to direct me in these Descriptions, and to make them as clear and intelligible as might be.

I was discouraged, upon first thinking of this Work, at the great Expence of graving, printing, and other things, which I knew would be a certain Cost attended with a very uncertain Profit, till my good Friend Mr. Catesby put me on etching my Plates myself, as he had done in his Works; and not only so, but invited me to see him work at Etching, and gave me all the necessary Hints and Instructions to proceed, which Favour I think myself obliged publickly to acknowledge. When I had practised a little while, I resolved to do such new and uncommon Birds, as I had in my Possession, since I saved Expences and only employed my Time.

In etching Plates which are afterwards to be coloured, I have discovered, that they should be done in a manner different from such things that are to continue Black and White; therefore I am willing to publish such Remarks on that Head, as may perhaps be of use to others that may hereafter publish any thing of that kind. He who would make a Print after any coloured Drawing, should make his Lights much lighter than they are in the Drawing, and the Shadows rather darker, which will indeed give your Print a somewhat shocking degree of Light and Shadow; but when you consider that by colouring, your Lights will become darker, and your very black Shadows, by being washed with Colours, which generally are lighter than Black, will become something lighter; in Prints for colouring it will be convenient to leave pretty broad clean white places that are a little dark in your colour'd Drawing: For Example, if a Part in your Drawing be of Blue or Red, or any fine Colour pretty deep; if you make your Print of so deep a Shade in those Parts, the Blackness will cast through the transparent Colours which you must use in washing Prints, and render them dead and dirty; and if you lay on too great a body of Colour, it will darken your Figure too much in the

Lights,

Lights, and make it flat and heavy. On the contrary, if you leave Lights as broad and as clean as the thing will permit, your Colours laid on such light Parts will appear with more Lustre than with black Strokes under them; and when the Print is washed with a little Judgment, it will lose its too great Proportion of Light and Shadow, and become soft and agreeable, and deceive tolerable Judges so far as to pass for a Water-colour'd Drawing. Prints that are not worked with a direct Design for colouring, cannot so easily be brought to that Beauty; they must be labour'd and painted with body Colours to make them look tolerably.

I do not purpose to part with any of the Prints uncolour'd while I live, lest they should be afterwards colour'd by unskilful People, which might be a Blemish to the Work, by being seen and taken for my Colourings. A Copy carefully and exactly colour'd from the original Drawings, will be deposited in the Library of the College of Physicians, *of* London, *which may serve as a Standard to refer to and compare with, to try the Truth of the Colouring, in case the Plates should outlive me, and any should question the Authority of the Colouring. I had thought when I first set out on this Work to have graved One hundred Plates of new Birds, but found I was under a necessity to leave off at Fifty, not being able to procure any more but such as have been described by many others. Seeing it is now known that I have done these, and am willing to go on, if I can procure any more of curious Gentlemen, I hope such Gentlemen of Taste this way, who have at any time Birds new and curious, will please to give me notice, that I may wait on them to take Drawings, which Favours I shall always gratefully acknowledge. It is now my duty to acknowledge, with all possible Gratitude, the Assistance I have received from many curious Gentlemen, and give my publick Thanks in general for the many and great Favours I have received from these my honourable and worthy Patrons and Friends, who from time to time have given me free Access to their Houses, and intrusted me in their Cabinets of Curiosities, and have oftentimes lent me very valuable and curious Things in order to forward me in my Pursuits: Yet in the course of these Descriptions I for my own Reputation (in order to prove the Being of the Birds here represented) have mentioned the Names in particular of my Patrons,*

Patrons, Friends, and others, who were the Poffeffors of thefe things, that I might have no opportunity to impofe Falfhood on the World, without being contradicted by living Witneffes.

I have made the Drawings of thefe Birds directly from Nature, and have, for variety's fake, given them as many different Turns and Attitudes as I could invent: This I chofe the rather to do, becaufe I know great Complaint hath been made, that a late Writer on Birds had given his Birds no variety of Pofture, but that they were direct Profiles ftanding in the fame Pofition, which famenefs is difagreeable. I obferved alfo in his Trees, Stumps, and Grounds, a poornefs of Invention; therefore to amend that Part in mine, I have taken the Counfel and Affiftance of fome Painters my particular Friends, in order to make the Work not only as natural and agreeable as I could in the fubject Matter, but to decorate the Birds with airy Grounds, having fome little Invention in them: The better to fet off the whole, I have in a few Plates, where the Birds were very fmall, added fome foreign Infects to fill up the naked Spaces in the Plates; thefe I efteem no part of the propofed Work, neverthelefs I have been equally careful to be exact in them both as to the Drawing and Colouring. Great part of the Birds, defcribed in this Work, were living when I drew them; others were in Cafes well preferved and dry, and fome were kept in Spirits, which is the better way to preferve them, tho' they cannot be fo well drawn in Spirits, by reafon the Forms of the Glaffes alter the apparent Shapes of the Birds; therefore I took fuch Birds out of the Spirits.

In the following Defcriptions I had a View, particularly in defcribing the Colours, to exprefs myfelf in fuch Terms as the Prints might be tolerably colour'd for the future by any curious obferving Perfon from the Defcriptions only, for in that refpect I have been as careful as I could, always comparing the Colours I mention to fome well-known thing when I could do it; and where I could not, I have ufed compound Terms, fuch as yellowifh Brown, redifh Brown, dirty Brown, and the like; and to other Colours I have added faint, dark, middling, inclining to this, that, or the other Colour: all which things are very neceffary in Natural Hiftory; for the fimple Terms Red, Blue, Yellow, &c. fignify a vaft Number of different Colours.

I fhall

*I shall presently conclude this Preface, and hope the Reader will excuse
its Length. As I never till very lately had any design to appear in
Print, I have neglected to study the Art of writing correctly, and am
sensible of the many Faults that may be found in this Book; but hope the
candid Reader will overlook them, since my chief Aim was rather to be
understood, than to write correctly.*

G. E.

A D D E N D A.

THE following Accounts are taken out of *Voyages*, and relate
to the *King of the Vultures*, Page 2 of this Book; and they coming to hand after the Descriptions were printed, I have placed them here.

Navarette in his Voyages in *Spanish*, Page 300, mentions *Rey de les
Zopilotes*, translated in *Churchill's Collection of Voyages*, Vol. 1. Page 235,
where he says, " That at *Acapulco* he saw the *King of the Zopilotes*,
" which are the same we call *Vultures*, it is one of the finest Birds
" that may be seen. I have often heard it prais'd, and, as I thought,
" they over-did it; but when I saw the Creature, I thought the De-
" scription far short of it."

Navarette in another Place of the above Translation, Page 46. speaks
thus: " But the gayest and finest Bird I have seen, is the *King of the*
" *Copilotes*, which I saw several times in the Port of *Acapulco*, and never
" had enough of looking at him, still more and more admiring his
" Beauty, Stateliness and Grace." This *Spanish* Author has used *z* and
c indifferently in the beginning of the Name, they sounding equally
and meaning the same Bird.

Sir *Hans Sloane* favour'd me with these Remarks, and we think, that
they can relate to no other Bird but the *King of the Vultures* described
in Page 2. What is now mentioned may serve pretty certainly to fix
his native Place, which before we did not know.

The

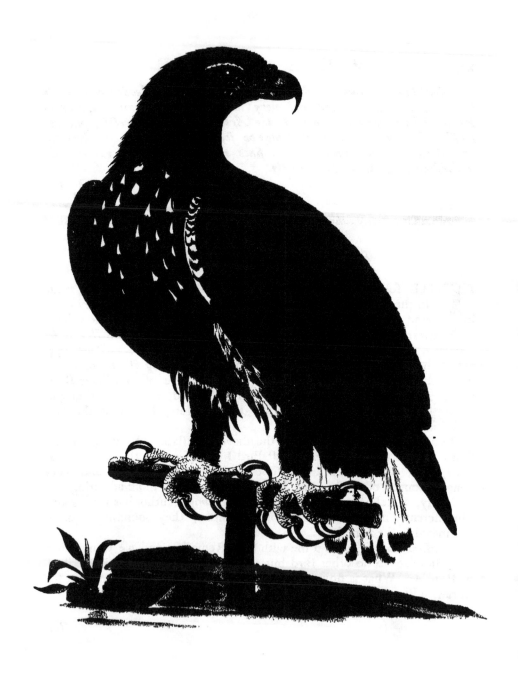

The WHITE TAILED EAGLE.

THIS Bird not agreeing, in all Refpects, with any of the Eagle-kind hitherto defcribed, and coming from a Part of the World we know but little of, I have given it a Place here. It is of the common Size of *Eagles*, that is about the bignefs of a *Cock-Turkey*. For Shape, it is flat-crown'd, fhort-neck'd, full-breafted, and brawny-thigh'd, having very long and broad Wings, in Proportion to the Body. The Bill is of a bluifh, Horn-colour, the upper Mandible arch'd, and hanging over the lower, about an Inch, having an Angle or Tooth on each Side· The lower Mandible is fhorter than the Upper, and received into it, the upper Mandible is covered about a third of its Length, from the Head, with a yellow Skin, called the *Cera*, from its refembling Wax, in which the Noftrils are fituate: This yellow Skin reaches on both Sides, quite round the Corners of the Mouth The Iris of the Eye is of a Hazel-colour; the Pupil, black, as it is in all Birds I have yet feen: Wherefore this Obfervation need not be repeated in the Sequel of this Work. Between the Bill and the Eyes, are Spaces of bare Skin, of a dirty Colour, thinly fet with fmall, black Hairs· The Head and Neck are covered with narrow, brown Feathers, ending in fharp Points, like thofe on the Necks of *Cocks*, but not fo long in Proportion: The whole Body is cover'd with dusky, brown Feathers, darker on the Back, and lighter on the under Side. The Breaft is fpotted with white, triangular Spots, having the fharpeft Angles pointing upwards: Thefe Spots are in the middle of each Feather. The covert Feathers of the Wings are of the Colour of the Body; the Quills, or Flag-feathers of the Wings, are black: A few of the Quills, and firft Row of Coverts, next the Back, are variegated with tranfverfe Lines, of a darker and lighter Colour. The Tail, which is of equal Length with the Wings, when clofed, is white, both upper and under Surface, except the Tips of the Feathers, which are black or dark brown; and the covert Feathers under the Tail, are of a redifh brown, or bay Colour; the Thighs are covered with dark, brown Feathers, of a very loofe Texture, through which a white Down appears in fome Places; the Legs are covered quite down to the Feet, with foft Feathers of a redifh, brown Colour. It hath four Toes on each Foot, very thick and ftrong, covered with Scales of a yellow Colour, ftanding three forward, and one backward, after the ufual Manner, armed with very ftrong Talons or Claws, of a black Colour, bending almoft into femicircular Figures, ending in very fharp Points.

This *Eagle* is a Native of *Hudfon's-Bay*, in the northern Part of *America*, from whence it was brought by a Gentleman, employ'd in the *Hudfon's-Bay* Company's Service, and by him prefented to my very good Friend, Dr. *R. M. Maffey*, who obliged me with a Sight of it. He kept it many Years at his Houfe at *Stepney*, near *London*, where I made the Drawing, from which this Print was taken.

B

The

The KING *of the* VULTURES.

THIS Bird is about the Bigneſs of a *Hen-Turkey*. I believe it is ſomething leſs than the greater Sort of *Vultures*; nor has it ſuch large Wings in Proportion. The Bill is pretty thick and ſtrong, ſtraight for a little way, then bends into a Hook, and over-hangs the lower Mandible, it is red at the Point, and black in the middle Part; the Baſe of the Bill, both upper and lower Mandibles, are cover'd with a Skin of an orange Colour, broad, and pointing to the Crown of the Head, on each Side above, in which Spaces are placed the Noſtrils, of an oblong Shape Between the Noſtrils is a looſe flap of Skin, ſcolloped, which falls indifferently on either Side of the Bill, when the Bird moves its Head. The Iris of the Eye is of a bright, pearly Whiteneſs; round the Eye, is an indifferent broad ſpace of Scarlet Skin, the Head and Neck are cover'd with bare Skin; the Crown of a dirty, Fleſh-colour, toward the Bill, and Scarlet in the hinder Part, behind which is a little Tuft of black Hairs From this Tuft proceeds, on each Side, and parts the Head from the Neck, a ſort of Stay of wrinkled Skin, of a browniſh Colour, with a little Blue and Red in its hinder Part: The Sides of the Head are of a black or dirty Colour, with Spots of browniſh Purple behind the Angles of the Mouth; the Sides of the Neck are red, which gradually becomes yellow in its fore Part; there runs a dirty yellow Liſt down the hind Part of the Neck; and at the bottom of the Neck, a Ruff of looſe, ſoft, aſh-colour'd Feathers, quite round, in which, by Contraction, it can hide its whole Neck and Sides of the Head, the Breaſt, Belly, Thighs, and covert Feathers under the Tail are White, or a little inclining to Cream-colour, the back and upper Part of the Wings is of a light, rediſh brown, inclining to Buff-colour, the Rump and upper covert Feathers of the Tail are White, the Quill-feathers of the Wings, black; ſome of the middle-moſt Quills have their Shafts edged with white; the Row of Coverts, next above the Quills, is black, with light, brown Edges; the Tail is wholly black, tho' Mr. *Albin* makes it black only at the End, the Legs and Feet are of a dirty, white Colour, the forward Toes are joined a little way by a Membrane; the Claws are black, not ſo great nor crooked as in Eagles.

This Bird I drew at Sir *Hans Sloane*'s, where it lived ſome Years. I have ſeen three or four of them; but could diſcover no ſuch Craw of bare Skin, as *Albin* has figured. The People who made a Shew of this Bird in *London*, told me it was brought from the *Eaſt Indies*, tho' I believe it rather to come from the *Weſt*. I have ſeen an old *Dutch* Print of this Bird, very incorrect, intitled, *Rex Warwouwarum, ex India Occidentali* Mr. *Perry*, a great Dealer in foreign Birds and Beaſts, has aſſured me theſe Birds are brought only from *America*. *Albin* ſuppoſes it to be like the *Braſilian Vulture*, called, *Urubu, Willoughby, p. 68*. tho' it differs widely from that which is no other than the *Turkey Buzard*, deſcribed in *Cateſby*'s Hiſtory of *Carolina*. Had Mr *Albin* been tolerably correct in his Figure of this Bird, I ſhould not have publiſhed a ſecond Draught.

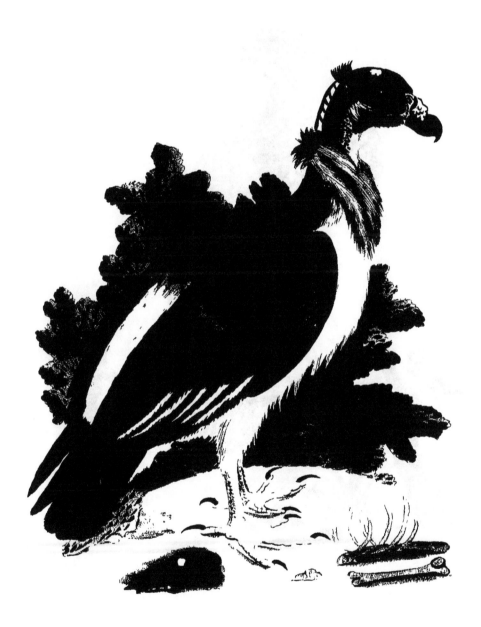

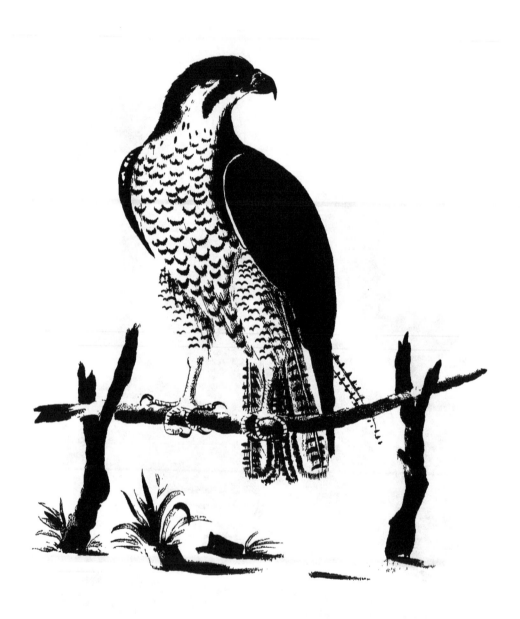

The SPOTTED HAWK *or* FALCON.

THIS Bird is of the Bigness of a common *Crow*, as near as I could judge, and well shaped, the Head being pretty small and sharp; the Neck, short, the upper Part of the Body pretty round, and falls tapering to a Narrowness downward; the Train pretty long, and the Wings reaching almost to the End thereof, the Thighs, muscular and strong, the Legs of middling Length, the Toes connected by a Membrane a little way, the Bill is hooked, and bent downward, having an Angle in the upper Mandible, into which the lower or shorter is received. The Base of the upper Mandible is covered with a Skin, in which are placed the Nostrils. The Bill is of a Lead-colour, the Cera of a greenish Yellow, the Skin at the Corners of the Mouth of a redish Yellow, the Iris of the Eye is of a dark Colour, round the Eye is a bare Space of Lead-colour'd Skin; the Top of the Head, Neck, Back, and upper Side of the Wings, are of a middling brown Colour, the under Side from the Bill to the Tail, is white, spotted in the Throat with little dashes, of a dark Colour, tending downward, which gradually change their Shape into the Form of Crescents, finer on the Breast, more gross on the Belly. The Thighs are spotted with smaller Spots, which may be better conceived by the Figure than described in Words. The Quills, and the Row of Feathers immediately above them, are painted with transverse Lines of black or dusky; the upper Part of the Ridge of the Wing which cover the Breast is white, the covert Feathers within-side of the Wings are dusky, spotted with round Spots of white, from the corners of the Mouth under the Eyes, on each Side, is drawn a broad, black Mark, which tends downward as far as the beginning of the Neck. The Rump and upper Side of the Tail is of a dark Ash-colour, with transverse Lines of Black. The under Side of the Tail and Quill-feathers are of a lighter Ash-colour, and the Bars that cross them, fainter than in the upper, the Legs and Feet of a bright Yellow, covered with a scaley Skin, the Toes are armed with strong, sharp-pointed, black Claws, pretty much bent. I shall not, in the Course of this Work, trouble the Reader with the Number and Situation of the Toes, the Figures plainly expressing them, yet I shall describe all such as have not the usual Number, or whose Toes stand not in the ordinary Position.

This Bird was brought from *Hudson's-Bay*, and presented to Dr. *Massey* at *Stepney*, where it lived some short Time. This Draught was taken while the Bird was alive.

The

The BLACK HAWK *or* FALCON.

THIS *Falcon* or *Hawk* (for I take it, that these two Names should import the same thing, tho' it is usual to give the Name of *Falcon* to those of the greater Kind, and such only as are trained for Sport, the lesser Sort being generally call'd *Hawks*) is of the same Magnitude with that immediately foregoing, and in all Respects shaped like it, excepting that it is a little bigger-headed in proportion to the Body : The Bill is of a dark Lead-colour, a little inclining to Flesh-colour, the Skin covering it of the same Colour, but a little more inclining to Yellow ; the Eye is of a dark Colour, with a bare Skin of a light Lead-colour round it, the Eyebrows overhang the Eyes, and are of a red Colour; the upper Side of the Head, Neck, Back, Wings and Tail, are of a black or very dark, dusky Colour : The Tips of the covert Feathers of the Wings and Tail are a little russet or redish ; it is also a little redish in the hinder Part of the Neck: The Ridge of the Wing in the upper Part is white, the Quills within-side, are marked with transverse Bars of dusky and Clay colour, as is the under Side of the Tail; the inner Coverts of the Wings are black, with round and irregular white Spots, the whole under Side is of a dirty Clay-colour, with black Spots at the Ends of the Feathers, in the Form expressed in the Figure. It hath black Marks from the Corners of the Mouth on each Side, extended backward in the form of Whiskers ; round these black Marks is a small Mixture of dusky White ; the Legs and Feet are of a dirty, greenish Lead-colour, but inclining more to Yellow, where the Legs and Feet join ; the Soles of the Feet redish, the Claws black.

This Bird is a Native of *Hudson's-Bay* · It pitched on a Ship belonging to the *Hudson's-Bay* Company in *August* 1739, as the Ship was returning Home, after they had got a pretty Way through the Straits to Sea, and lived in *London* all the hard Winter, 1739. I was favour'd with a Sight of this Bird by *Taylor White*, Esq; who gave me Liberty to draw it. Whether this and the foregoing be Male and Female, I leave to the Judgment of those who understand Natural History.

The

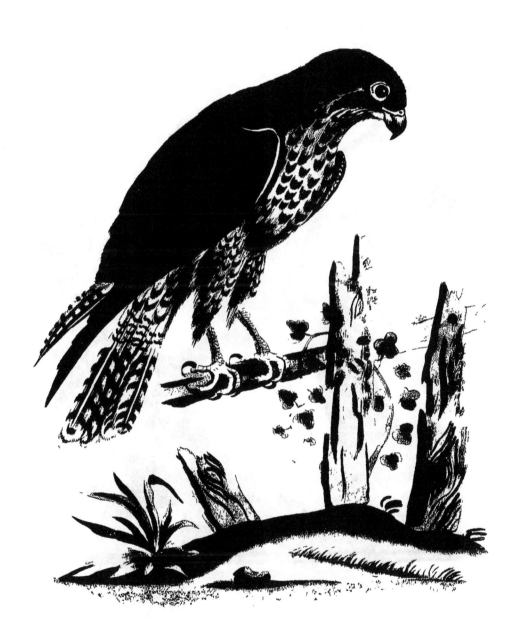

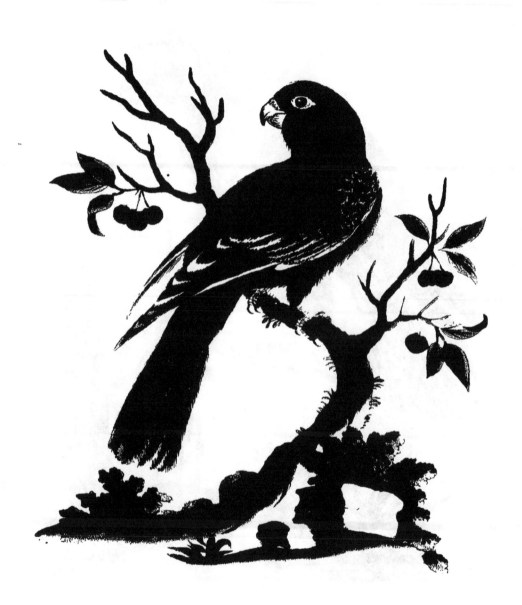

The BLACK PARROT *from* Madagascar.

THIS Bird is about the Bignefs of the Afh-colour'd *Parrot* with a red Tail, or a *Tame Pigeon*. The Bill is fhort and thick at the Bafis, bending downward as an Arch, the lower Mandible bending in the fame manner upwards; the upper Mandible over-hangs the lower a little, but much lefs than I have obferved it in fome other *Parrots :* The Bafis of the upper Mandible is covered with a bare Skin, in which are fituate the Noftrils, pretty high and near each other; both the Bill and the Skin that covers it, were white, or light, yellowifh, Flefh-colour; the Eyes had dark Irides, and a Space of bare white Skin round them: The Head and whole Body, both upper and under Side, is of a black or very dark, dirty, bluifh Colour, like the Colour of *Pigeons*, which we call *Black Pigeons*, not like the Black of *Crows :* The upper Side of the Wings is lighter, being only of a dark, Afh-colour; amongft the Quill-feathers are intermixed three or four white Feathers in each Wing; the Feathers of the Wings are pretty long; the Tail is very long, for one whofe Tail-feathers are of equal Length as this is, they having generally very fhort Tails; that kind of *Parrots*, whofe Tail-feathers are of un-equal Lengths, are as remarkable for very long Tails; the Legs are very fhort, and the Toes fituate two backward and two forward, as in all the *Parrot*-kind; they are cover'd with a rough, fcaley Skin, of a dirty Flefh-colour; the Claws are ftrong, crooked and black.

This Bird was firft Sir *Charles Wager*'s, and was prefented by him to his Grace the Duke of *Richmond*, who employ'd me to make a Draught of it for him, and permitted me to take another for myfelf. It was a very gentle Bird, always choofing to be on the Hand, and when taken on the Hand, it would often repeat the Act of Treading, which makes me think it was a Cock-Bird. I believe it hath not yet been defcribed.

C

The smallest GREEN *and* RED INDIAN PAROQUET.

IN this Plate, which was wrought from Nature, and not from a Drawing, the Bird is represented of its proper Size. It is less than the small red-headed *Paroquet*, commonly brought into *England*, which is pretty well figur'd and describ'd by *Albin* in his History of Birds, *Vol.* 3. *Page* 15. tho' his Drawing is something too small, seeing the Bird is a little bigger than what I have here represented, which is the least of the *Parrot*-kind I ever met with; the Bill is shaped like those in the greater Sort of *Parrots*, of a bright Orange-colour. I could perceive no Skin covering the Basis of the Bill; the Nostrils were near together in the upper Part of the Bill, very near the Feathers of the Forehead; the Eyes are surrounded with a narrow Space of Skin, of a light Flesh-colour; the Top of the Head is Red, or of the Colour of a *Sevil* Orange, which in the hinder Part of the Head gradually becomes Green, uniting itself with the Colour of the Back; the under Side of the Bird, middle of the Back, Wings, and Tail, are of a fine Green-colour, lighter on the Throat, Breast, Belly, and Thighs, and darker on the Back Coverts of the Wing and Tail, darkest of all in the greater Wing-feathers; the lower Half of the Back and Rump, quite to the Tail, is covered with the same bright Red or Orange-colour with the Head, being intermixed with the Green, and losing itself in the middle of the Back; the Legs, Feet, and Claws, are of a Flesh-colour, the Toes standing as in other *Parrots*; the inside of the Quills, and the under-side of the Tail are Blue a very little inclining to Green.

This Bird was brought from *Holland*, in Spirits, by Dr. *Cromwell Mortimer*, Secretary to the *Royal Society*, who bought it there with other Things brought from some *Dutch* Settlement in the *East Indies*. He was pleased to lend it me, that I might draw it. This Bird was put in camphorated Spirits, and appeared of a brown Colour whilst in the Spirits, tho' the Glass was white Flint, and the Spirits clear; and when taken out, washed and dried, it became of the Colours above described. I believe no Author hath yet taken notice of this Bird.

The

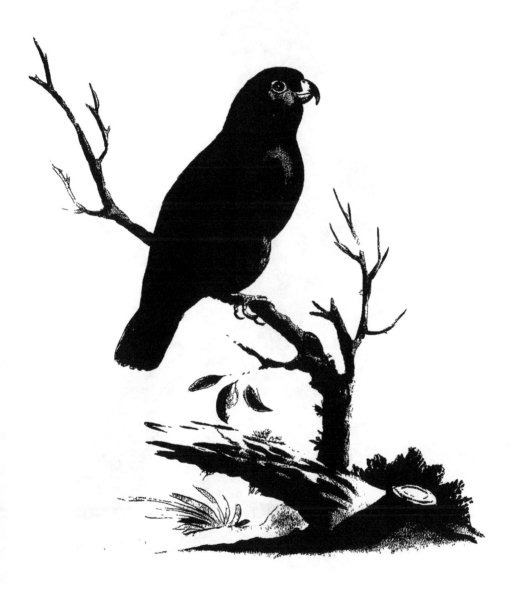

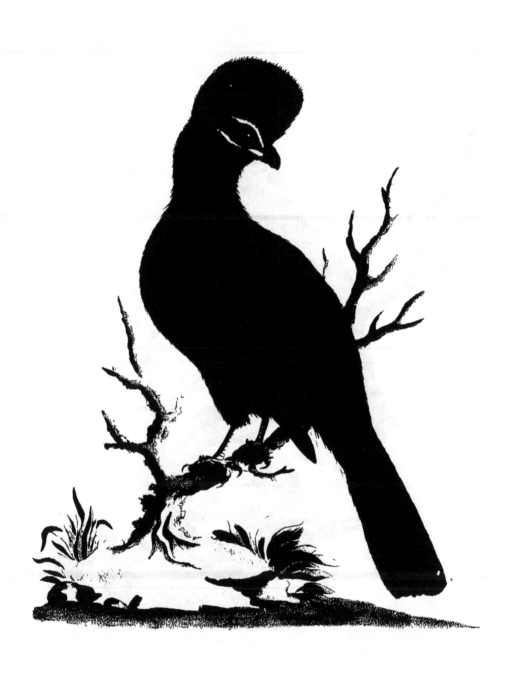

The TOURACO.

THIS Bird is about the Bigness of a *Magpye* or *Jay*, the Make of its Body is rather long than round, the Head of a moderate Size, the Neck of a middling Length; the Legs rather short than long; the Tail pretty long: It is a very elegant Bird, both for Shape and Colour, it is very active, slurting up its Tail, and raising its Crest, it swells its Throat, and utters a hoarse and disagreeable Sound, the Bill is short and compressed Side-ways, the upper Mandible a little arched, but not over-hanging the lower; the under Side of the lower Mandible has a small Angle, as in the Bills of *Gulls*, the upper and lower Chaps are of a dirty Red or Brick Colour· I know not any Bird that has a Bill like this. The Eye is of a dark Hazel-colour, encompassed with a knotty Skin of a bright Scarlet-colour, from the Corner of the Mouth to the Eye, is a broad black Line, which grows narrower, and extends itself under and beyond the Eye; under this is a white Line, which extends a little farther back than the black Line, but doth not come forward so near the Bill, from the Corner of the Mouth is extended another white Line, which passes above the Eye, but not so far back as that beneath; the Head, Neck, Breast, and lesser Coverts of the Wings, are of a fine dark, Green-colour; on its Head it hath a Crest, which it raiseth at Pleasure, the very Tips of the Feathers on the Crest are Red; the Thighs, lower Belly, and Coverts under the Tail, are dusky or black, the Back, Wings, and Tail, are of a fine bluish Purple-colour, part of the greater Wing-feathers or Quills, next the Belly, are of a fine Crimson-colour, well expressed by pure Carmine, their Tips and Borders of the outer Webs are black; the Legs, Feet, and Claws, Ash-colour, the Toes are situate as in *Woodpeckers*, *Parrots*, and *Cuckows* What Genus of Birds to range this with, I cannot positively say; it climes not as *Parrots* do, nor doth it agree with them in any respect, except in the Position of the Toes; nor is its Bill any thing like a *Woodpecker's*, so that I think it nearest the *Cuckow*-kind. *Albin* has figur'd this Bird, and calls it the *Crown Bird* from *Mexico*, tho' these Birds are indeed *Africans*, brought from *Guinea*, by the Way of the *West Indies*, to us, he hath not shaped his Bill right, nor described well the Marks about the Eye, he mentions White in the Wings, which I could not discover, tho' I have drawn after two different Birds of this Kind

This Bird is now living at Colonel *Louther*'s House in St. *James's* Park, where I have been permitted to make Drawings of it for several Persons of Distinction. The Texture of this Bird's Feathers are so fine, that no distinct Form of Feathers can be discovered, except in the Wings and Tail. See Mr *Albin*'s Figure, *Vol.* 2, *Page* 18. of his *Natural History of Birds*. His Bird was either a great deal less than mine, or one of us must be pretty much mistaken in the Size, since he makes it of the Size of the *Missel* Bird, which is not above half the Bigness of a *Jay* or *Magpye*, to which I have likened it for Size.

The

The GREAT KING-FISHER *from the River* Gambia.

FOR Bignefs, this Bird equals, if not exceeds, the *Miffel* Bird or *Greater Thrufh*; it is great-headed, fhort-necked, the Body neither over-long or round, the Tail is long, the Wings pretty long, the Legs very fhort; the Bill is long and ftraight, pretty thick towards the Head, ending in a fharp Point, of a bright Scarlet-colour; the upper Mandible is channelled on each Side, in which Channels are placed the Noftrils, pretty near the Head; the Angles or Corners of the Mouth are deep cut, and fall directly under the Eyes; under each Eye is a narrow Border of white Feathers; the Head, Neck, whole under Side, and part of the Back, are cover'd with dirty Orange-colour'd Feathers; the Chin and Breaft lighter than the Back; in the Middle of the Breaft, some of the Tips of the Feathers are White; the Wings are Purple, in the upper Part the greater Feathers being Blue, yet the foremoft of the prime Quills are Black; tho' the upper Part of the Wing be moftly Purple, yet there is a narrow Space of Blue runs round the Purple; the Ridge of the Wing is White; the lower Part of the Back and Rump is of a Blue-Green, changeable Colour; the Wing-feathers, which border on the Back, partake of the fame changeable Colour; the Tail is of a fine Blue-colour, yet it in fome Lights has a greenifh Caft; the Legs and Feet are of a Red-colour, with black Claws; the middle and outer Toe joined together, as in our *King-fifher*. This Bird was preferv'd in the Collection of Mr. *Peter Colinfon*, who on all Occafions has been my Friend, and helped me to many curious and uncommon Birds: He told me this Bird came from the River *Gambia*.

Albin has publifhed a Bird fomething like this, which he calls the *Large King-fifher* from *Bengal*; but there is fo much Difference, that they muft be two different Species: I have feen both the Birds; *Albin's* is in Mr. *Dandridge's* Collection in *Moorfields*, which has convinced me they are fpecifically different, more than if I had feen only Drawings of thefe two Birds. See *Albin's* Figure and Defcription, *Vol.* 3. *p.* 27. of his *Hiftory of Birds*.

The

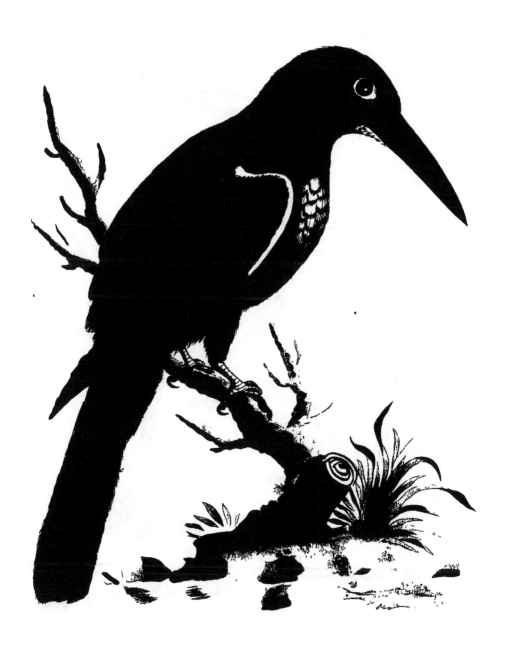

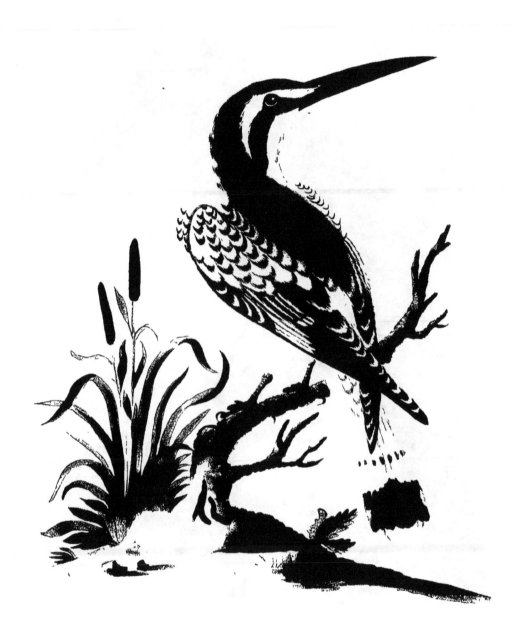

The BLACK and WHITE KING-FISHER.

THIS Bird is of the Bigneſs of the *Song Thruſh*, the Figure is of the natural Size; it hath a long ſtraight Bill, flat Crown, long Head, and ſhort Neck; the Head, I think, not ſo big in proportion to the Body, as in ſome others of this Genus; it hath pretty long Wings, and a long Tail; all of the *Kings-fiſher*-kind are ſhort-leg'd; the Bill is long and pretty thick at the Baſe, ending in a ſharp Point, of a black Colour, having a Groove or Channel on each Side the upper Mandible, in which the Noſtrils are placed near the Baſe; the Eyes are placed juſt over the Corners of the Mouth; the Crown of the Head and hinder Part of the Neck is black; from the Corners of the Mouth, under the Eyes, is a broad black Line, which falls into the ſame Colour behind the Neck; from the Noſtrils are drawn white Lines above the Eyes, and continued the whole Length of the Head; the whole under Sides, from Bill to Tail, is of a dirty, yellowiſh White, except a little Bar of black Spots that croſſes the Middle of the Breaſt; the whole Back is black, the Feathers having grey Tips; the Ridge of the Wing is White; all the Covert-feathers party-colour'd of Black and White; the baſtard Wing Black; the firſt or largeſt Quill-feathers are white at their Bottoms, then black, having the very Tips white; the middle Quills have white Spots in their outer Webs, and white Tips; the remaining Quills next the Back, are black with white Tips; the Tail-feathers are white toward their Bottoms, with a Row of tranſverſe black Spots; toward the Tips is a Bar of Black of an Inch broad, the Tips beyond the Bar being White; the Legs and Feet are of a dirty brown Colour, ſhap'd as in all others of this Kind. Mr *Peter Colinſon* lent me this Bird to draw; he received it with others from *Gamron* in *Perſia*.

This Bird was preſerv'd in Spirits, with many others, in a Glaſs to bring to *England*, the white Part appeared very dirty and yellow, which, I believe, was owing only to its being ſtained with the foul Spirits, for I have obſerv'd ſuch Changes in Feathers which I knew otherwiſe to be purely White.

N. B. If any one would draw a Bird preſerv'd in Spirits, let him take it out, waſh it pretty well in warm Water, and rinſe it in a good Quantity of cold, and let it dry gradually, and he will reſtore the true Colour of the Feathers, as far as can be; for ſome Feathers in the Glaſſes of Spirits, I have obſerved to appear of Colours very contrary to the true Colour they are of before they were put in.

D

The

❋ *The* SWALLOW-TAIL'D KING-FISHER.

THIS Plate reprefents the Bird in its natural Size, which is nearly that of the *Englifh King-fifher*, and it agrees alfo with ours in Shape, except the Wing being a little longer, and the Tail much longer, without regard to the two longeft Feathers; the Bill is long, ftraight, and fharp-pointed, black of Colour, channeled on each Side in the upper Mandible, in which Channels are placed, the Noftrils pretty near the Head; the Corners of the Mouth fall deep into the Head, and the Eyes are placed juft over them; the Head is of a dirty brown Colour, brighter towards the Bill, darker in the hinder Part; under the Bill is a pretty large white Spot an Inch broad, in the middle Part, but growing narrower on each Side toward the Neck; the whole Body is of a dirty Black, having a glofs of Blue, fomething lighter on the Breaft, and darker on the Back; the Wings are of a fine, dark, fhining Green, tho' lighter in the Covert-feathers than in the Quills; a fingle white Feather appear'd among the Covert-feathers of the Wing; the Tail had two long Feathers more than double the Length of the other Feathers; the upper Side of a dark gloffy Green, on the under Side dusky, fome of the fhorter Feathers having white Tips; the Legs and Feet are Black, and made as in other *King-fifhers*. This Bird, tho' of a dull Colour, hath all over it, when expofed to the Sun, a fhining Luftre like a Mixture of Gold Threads with the Feathers, fuch as we fee in moft forts of *Huming Birds*; it is more remarkably bright on the Covert-feathers of the Wings than in any other Part.

This Bird is in his Grace the Duke of *Richmond*'s Collection; it was inclofed and pafted up in Glafs, fo that I could not handle it, nor could I certainly difcover whether the two long Feathers in the Tail were the middle Feathers or the outer Feathers; tho' I think they are the middle Feathers. The Bird we call *Merops* in *Europe*, differs from the *King-fifher*, only in that it hath the Bill a little bent downward, and the two middle Feathers of the Tail being longer than the reft; the Bird above defcribed, hath only one of thefe Marks of difference: It was brought from *Surinam* in *South America*, by the way of *Holland*. I cannot find that this Bird has been defcribed or taken notice of by any Author.

The

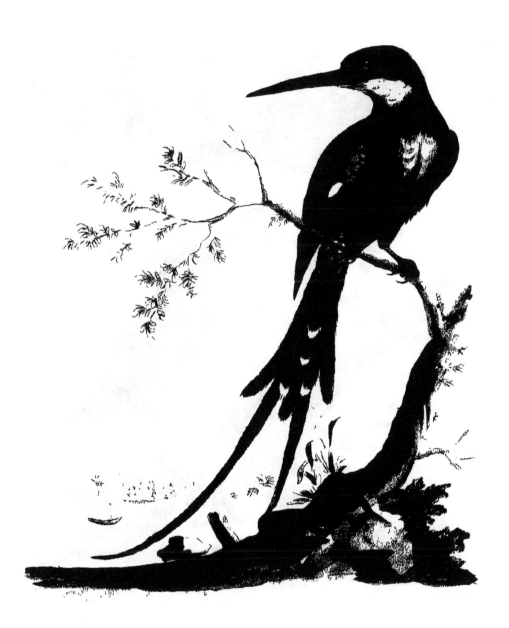

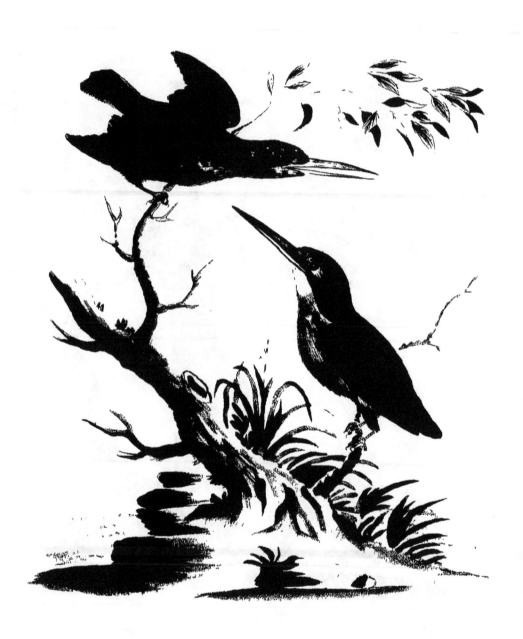

The little INDIAN KING-FISHERS.

THESE Birds fo nearly refemble the *King-fifher* we have in *England*, that the Defcription of the one will almoft anfwer for the other, except in the Bignefs, thefe being not half fo big as ours in *England*; the Plate fhews them in their natural Bignefs, there being fome fmall difference between thefe two Birds, it is like they may be Cock and Hen; the uppei Bird hath a yellow Bill, inclining to Orange; the whole under Side is of an Orange-colour; the Top of the Head, Neck, Back, Rump, and Covert-feathers of the Wings are Blue, the Points of the Feathers being very light and bright; at the Bafe of the upper Mandible of the Bill, on each Side, is an Orange-coloui'd Spot; behind each Ear likewife is a little Tuft of Oiange-coloui'd Feathers, which feem to ftand a little way out; the Feathers of the Tail, and all the Quills of the Wing, are of a dirty, blackifh Brown; the Legs and Feet are made as in other *King-fifhers*, of a dirty Orange-colour.

The lower Bird hath a black Bill, daiker towards the Point; the lower Chap for a little Space, next the Head, is Flefh-colour; the Throat is white; the Breaft, Belly, and whole under Side, is Orange-colour, tho' the Sides of the Belly are a little intermixed with Green; from the Noftrils, through the Eyes, are diawn on each Side, Lines of Orange-colour, which reaches down the Sides of the Neck; below thefe, on each Side from the Angles of the Mouth, are drawn Lines of Blue-green; the upper Side, Head, Neck, Back, Wings, and Tail, are cover'd with Blue-green Feathers; the Top of the Head and the Mark on the Cheek, has tranfverfe Lines of a darker Blue; the Tips of the Coverts of the Wings are lighter than the other Part of the Feathers; the Legs and Feet are of a dirty Red; the uppei Bird differs from our *King-fifher*, in that it hath a yellow Bill, which in ouis is black or dusky, and that this hath dirty brown Quill and Tail-featheis; ours are fo far edged with Green, as to appear Green when the Feathers are clofed. The lower Bird differs fiom ours, in not having veiy bright, blue Feathers on its Back and Rump, which in ouis aie remarkable foi their bright Luftre: Theie came with one of thefe Birds fiom *India* a *King fifher*, altogether like ouis in *England*, both for Bignefs, Shape, and Colour. Mr. *Peter Colinfon* obliged me with the upper Bird, and Mr. *Dandridge* with the lower. They came from *Bengal* in the *Eaft Indies*.

The

The ARABIAN BUSTARD.

THIS Bird is about the Bignefs of a *Turkey*, it is longer leg'd and neck'd, and flenderer-body'd than the common *Buftard* It hath a Bill longer than is common to the Poultry-kind, of which this is a Species From the Point of the Bill to the Angles of the Mouth is three Inches and a Half; the Bill is of a light Horncolour, a little darker at the Point; the Noftrils are long, and placed near the Forehead, the Eyes are of a dark Colour, the Fore-part of the Head is white, above the Eye is a Line of black, ending in a Point toward the Forehead backward, it increafes in Breadth, and forms a fort of black Creft, from which Creft proceeds a fhort black Line, and reaches almoft to the hinder Part of the Eye, the Neck, forward, is Afh-colour'd, with fmall tranfverfe Lines of a darker Colour, the hinder Part of the Neck and Back are of a brown Colour, with fine tranfverfe blackifh Lines, the Coverts of the Wings of the fame Colour with the Back, the Tips of the Feathers being white, form Spots like Half-moons; the Ridge of the Wing in the upper Part is White, from whence proceeds a broad white Bar, that feparates the Covert from the Quill-feathers, this Bar is fprinkled with fmall black Spots, few or none in the upper Part, thickly ftrewed in the lower, the baftard Wing is black, the Feathers having white Tips, the foremoft of the prime Quills are black, the middlemoft are fpotted black and white, being part of the above-mentioned Bar, drawn obliquely down the Wing, the inner Quills, next the Back, are of the fame Colour with it; the Breaft, Belly, Thighs, and whole under Side, are purely White, the Tail on the upper Side, is colour'd like the Back, tho' the outer Webs of the outfide Feathers are partly White, the under Side of the Tail hath a Bar of Black acrofs it, near the Tips of the Feathers; the Legs are pretty long; it has only three Toes, which are very fhort, all ftanding forward, the Legs are bare of Feathers for fome Space above the Knees, both Legs and Feet are cover'd with a fcaley Skin of a dirty white or light brownifh Colour; the Claws of the fame Colour.

This Bird was kept alive many Years by my honoured Patron Sir *Hans Sloane*, Bart. at his Houfe in *London*, whofe Goodnefs always gave me free Leave to draw any curious Thing he had in his Poffeffion. This Bird was brought from *Mocha* in *Arabia Felix*, and prefented to Sir *Hans Sloane*, by *Charles Dubois*, Efq, Treafurer to the *India* Company. It hath not yet been defcrib'd by any Author that I know of.

The

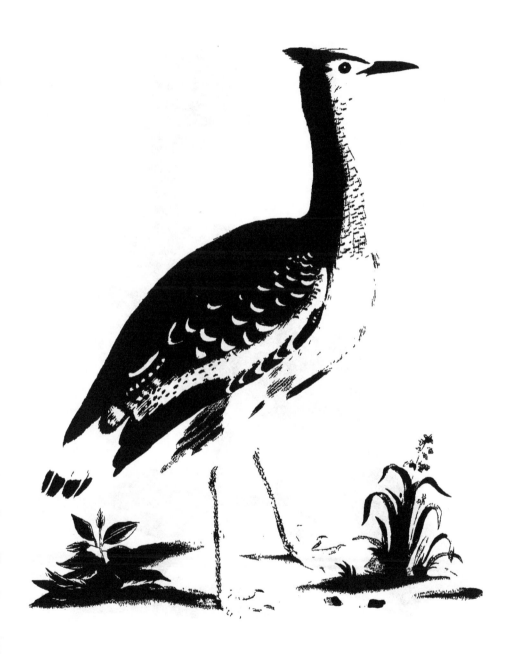

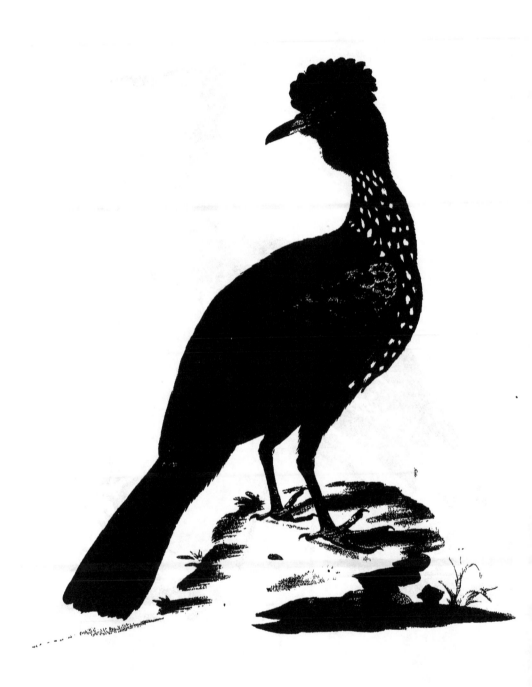

The QUAN *or* GUAN, *so called in the* Weſt Indies.

THIS Bird is a little bigger than a common *Hen*, near the Bigneſs of the larger Kind of Poultry; for Shape of Body, it pretty nearly reſembles a *Turkey*, to which I take it to be near of Kin; the Bill ſtraight, longer than a *Hen*'s Bill, bending down a little at the Point, of a black Colour; the Noſtrils placed pretty near the Head; the Sides of the Head are of a Blue-purple-colour'd Skin, bare of Feathers; in the middle of theſe bare Spaces are placed the Eyes, whoſe Irides are of a dark, dirty Orange-colour; under the Chin, and a little way down the Neck, there hangs a looſe Skin, of a fine red Colour, thinly ſet with black Hairs; the Top of the Head is cover'd with black Feathers, which it can erect into a Creſt; ſome have little or no Appearance of a Creſt, I ſuppoſe they are Hens; the whole Body, downward from the Head, is cover'd with black Feathers, or very dark, ruſty Brown; the fore-part of the Neck, Breaſt, and Belly, have white Spots and Daſhes tending downward, intermixed with the dark Colour; the Coverts of the Wings have ſomething of a green and purple Gloſs, the Quills more inclining to Purple; the Back and Rump reflect a Copper-colour'd Gloſs; but all theſe Gloſſes change to different Colours in different Poſitions of Light; yet in a bad Light, the Bird ſeems to be only of a ruſty Black, having no Luſtre at all; the Thighs and lower Belly are of a ruſty Black, having no Gloſs; the Tail is pretty long, ſhaped like a *Turkey*'s Tail, of a dull Black; the Legs and Feet are of a bright Red; it hath four Toes ſtanding after the uſual manner: I could ſee no Spurs it had; the three forward Toes are join'd together a little way by a Membrane; the Claws are black.

I ſaw one of theſe Birds at Captain *Chandler*'s at *Stepney*, who brought it with him from ſome one of the Sugar Iſlands in the *Weſt Indies*, I have forgot directly which; but I ſuppoſe it may be found in moſt of them. The *Braſilian Jacupema* of *Margrave*, I believe, is the ſame with this Bird, tho' his Deſcription differs ſomething from mine.

E

The GREEN-WING'D DOVE.

THIS *Dove* is reprefented in the Plate of its natural Bignefs: It is rather round than long-body'd; the Tail and Wings not fo long as in moft kind of *Doves.* I think it the moft beautiful of all the *Dove*-kind I have hitherto feen. The Bill is near an Inch long and pretty flender, of a Scarlet-colour, from the Point to the Noftrils, both upper and under Chaps; from the Noftrils to the Head of a pale Blue, a little Rifing in the upper Part; the Eye is of a dark Colour; the Forehead is white, from which proceed two white Lines above the Eyes, towards the hinder Part of the Head; the Crown of the Head is of a bluifh Colour; the Sides of the Head, Neck and Breaft, are of a Rofe-colour, tho' the hind Part of the Neck gradually changes to a more dirty Colour; the Belly is of a dirty Orange colour, which infenfibly foftens into and unites with the Rofe-colour of the Breaft; the upper Side of the Wings are of a fine Green-colour in fome Lights, which in other Pofitions to the Light, appear of a fplendid Copper-colour, or a Colour more inclining to Gold; the greater Quills are of a dirty Black; the Shoulder or Ridge of the Wing is fpotted with fmall white Spots; among the Covert-feathers of the Wing, on one Side only, was a fingle white Feather; the Sides, under the Wings, are of the fame Colour with the Belly; the Covert-feathers, within-fide of the Wings, are of a dark Cinnamon-colour; the inner Webs of the Quills from their Bottoms, for a good way towards their Tips, are alfo tinged of a Cinnamon-colour, other-wife they are of a dusky Black; the middle of the Back is of a dirty Brown; the lower Part of the Back, and the Feathers covering the Tail, are Afh-colour; the middle Feathers of the Tail are Black; the outer Feathers Afh-colour, with black Tips; the Legs and Feet are of a Red-colour, fuch as is common to moft of the *Pigeon*-kind; the Claws are light Brown.

This *Dove* was prefented to Mr. *John Warner,* Merchant in *Rotherhith,* at whofe Houfe I took a Draught of it. He told me it was brought from the *Eaft Indies.* I faw another of thefe Birds, kept fome time in a Cage at Sir *Hans Sloane*'s.

The

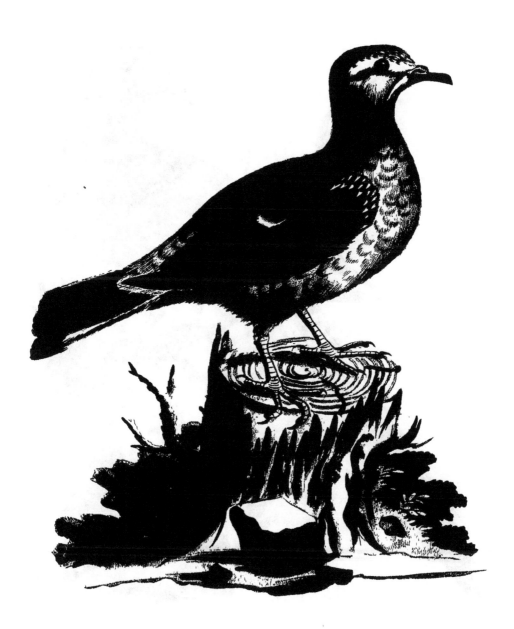

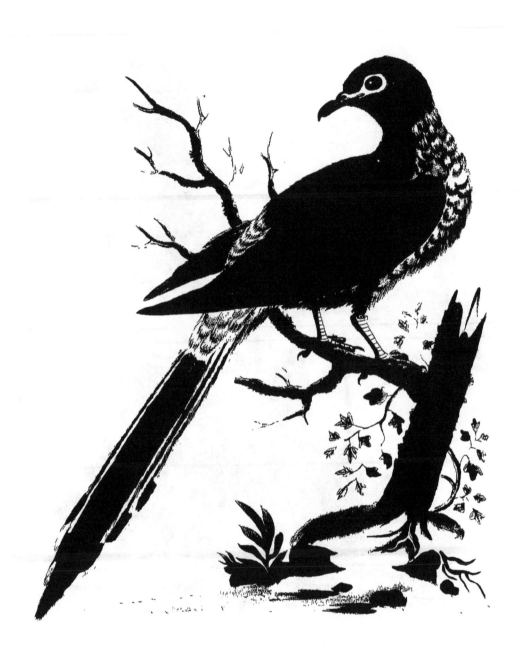

The LONG-TAIL'D DOVE.

THE Figure of this Bird fhews it of its natural Bignefs; it hath but a fmall Head in proportion to the Body, the Neck of a middling Length, the Body pretty long; the Tail longer than the whole Body, the Wings of middling Length, the Bill is ftraight, not very thick, a little bent downwards at the Point, of a Horn-colour, light about the Noftrils, and a little Rifing, darker towards the Point; the Iris of the Eye is of a dark Colour, from the Corner of the Bill to the Eye, is drawn a white Line, which incircleth the Eye, the Fore-part of the Head, above and beneath the Bill, is of a yellowifh or Clay-colour, the hinder Part is of a *Pigeon* Blue, pretty light, thefe Colours lofe themfelves in each other, where they unite, where thefe two Colours meet on the Sides of the Head, juft under the Ear-holes, are fituate on each Side a round black Spot of the bignefs of a Tare, the Fore-part of the Neck and Breaft are of a blufh or Bloffom-colour, more intenfe above, changing gradually to-wards the Belly into a Clay-colour, the lower Part of the Belly, Thighs, and Coverts under the Tail, being Clay-colour, with a little mixture of Cinerious, the upper Side of the Neck, Back, and upper Side of the Wings, is of a dark, dirty Brown, the Quills being darker than the Covert-feathers, though the Edges of the Webs of the Quill-feathers are a little lighter colour'd than the reft of the Wing, the Scapular-feathers between the Back and Wing, as alfo fome of the Quills and Coverts next the Back, are marked at their Ends with oval black Spots of different Magnitudes, about 10 or 12 in Number on each Side, the Rump, and Feathers covering the Tail, are more in-clining to Afh-colour than the Back and Wings, the middle Feathers of the Tail are very long and black, the fide Feathers gradually grow fhorter, fo that the outer-moft on each Side, little exceed half the Length of the middlemoft, the outer Feathers are of a bluifh or Afh-colour, having Bars of Black near their Tips, the Tips themfelves being White, the Legs and Feet Red, as in others *Doves*, it hath four Toes ftanding after the ufual Manner, the Claws are Brown What is moft fingular in this Bird, is the Length of the Tail, which is fhap'd like a *Magpye's*, no Bird of the *Dove* or *Pigeon*-kind, that I have met with, having the like This Bird hardly differs at all from fome others in the *Weft Indies*, fave in the Tail.

I drew this Bird at Mr *John Warnes's* of *Rotherhith*, who had it of a Perfon that brought it from the *Weft Indies*

The TRANSVERSE STRIPED *or* BARED DOVE.

THIS Bird for Shape, agrees with moft of the *Dove*-kind; for
Magnitude it is one of the fmaller Sort, being of the bignefs
of the Draught, or if any Difference, 'tis rather lefs; the Tail of a
pretty good Length, in Proportion to the Body, the Feathers being of
equal Length; the Bill is fhap'd as in other *Doves*, of a light Horn-
colour; from the Noftril to the Eye, and round the Eye, is a narrow
white Stroke; the Iris of the Eye, Blue-grey; the Forehead, round the
Eyes, Cheeks, and under the Bill, are light Blue; the Crown, and hinder
Part of the Head, are Red or Ruffet; the Fore-part of the Neck,
Breaft, Belly and Thighs, are of a faded Rofe or Bloffom-colour; the
Feathers under the Tail, White; the Sides of the Neck, and Sides of
the Body under the Wings, which partly appear when the Wings are
clofed, are of a bluifh Colour, thick fet with very fine tranfverfe Lines
of a darker Blue or Black; the upper Side of the Neck, Back, Wings
and Tail, are of a dirty, brownifh Afh-colour; the hinder Part of the
Neck, Back, and Covert-feathers of the Wings, are mark'd at little
Diftances with very diftinct tranfverfe Lines of Black, which are continued from Wing to Wing acrofs the Back, with little Breaks or Inter-
ruptions; the greater Quills are fomething darker than the Coverts of
the Wing: Though the Tail be of the Colour of the Body, yet the
outfide Feathers are darker, approaching to Black, having their Tips
White about an Inch deep; the Legs and Feet are fhap'd as in other
Doves, of a paler Red than is common to moft; the Claws brown.
Though I have mention'd many different Colours in this Bird, you muft
not underftand a fudden meeting of any two Colours, as in Patch-
work, but fuch an Union and gradual Change from one Colour to another, as a fkillful Painter expreffes in his fofteft Shadows.

I took this Draught from the Bird alive, at Sir *Charles Wager*'s Houfe
at *Parfons-Green*. I was told by Sir *Charles*'s Lady it was brought from
the *Eaft Indies*.

The

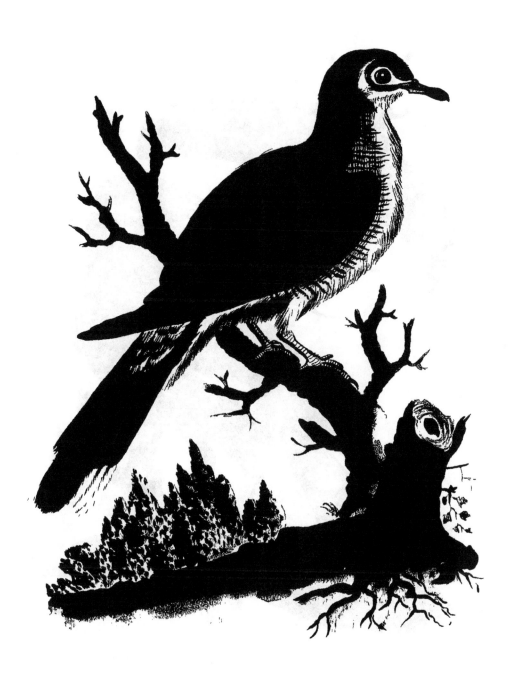

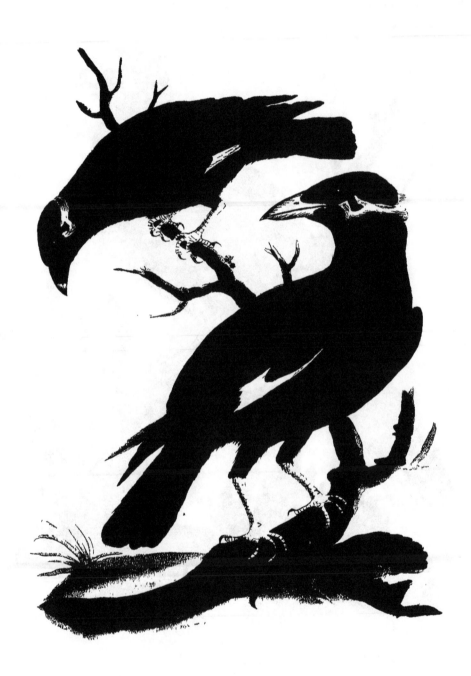

The MINOR *or* MINO, *Greater and Lefs.*

I Suppofe the above Name may be the *Indian* Name of this Bird, in the Country from whence it is brought. I take it to be near of Kin to the *Jacdaw*; the Greater, for Bignefs, equals a *Jackdaw* or *Magpye*, the Leffer hardly exceeds a *Black-Bird*, fo that the one is at leaft twice as big as the other; they have middling fiz'd Heads, pretty plump round Bodies, and fhort Tails; the Legs of a middling Length; the Bill is pretty thick at the Bafis, from upper to under Side, but fomething compreffed Sideways, of a red Colour towards the Head, and a yellow Point in the leffer Bird, and all over Yellow in the Greater, the Bill ends in a Point not very fuddenly or fharp; the Feathers on each Side point into the Bill as far as the Noftrils, the Eyes are Hazel-colour'd in both, in the hinder-part of the Head in both, are two little Flaps of yellow Skin in the form of Crefcents with the Points upwards, one Corner of each being behind the Eyes, the other Corners uniting in the hinder-part of the Head; under the Eyes are other yellow bare Spots of Skin, which are joined to the before-mention'd, in a manner not eafy to exprefs, but by the Figure, I have been more full in this Particular, becaufe Mr. *Albin* has publifhed this Bird, and falfly defcrib'd thefe Marks, which are the Characterifticks, both in his Figure and Defcription I have had opportunity to examine feveral of thefe Birds, tho' they are very rare The Head, Neck, whole Body, Wings and Tail, are cover'd with black Feathers of a great Luftre, fhining in different Lights with blue, green and purple Gloffes, the Feathers on the hinder-part of the Head, that are encompafs'd by the bare Flaps of Skin, refemble Hairs or Velvet for their Finenefs, the Bottoms of fome of the firft of the Quills are white, which form a white Spot in the middle of the Wing, the Legs and Feet are of a yellow Colour inclining to Orange in the leffer Bird, more Yellow in the Greater, the Claws light Brown; the Number and Pofition of the Toes, as in the Figure.

The leffer Bird I faw at a Dealer's in curious Birds, in *White-Hart Yard* in the *Strand*, *London*. The Greater, belong'd to the late Dr. *George Wharton*, Treafurer of the *College of Phyficians, London*, who employ'd me to draw it for his Lady, and gave me leave to take a Draught for myfelf. After it died, I open'd it and fet up the Skin I found it to be a Hen Bird. Whether thefe two Birds, fo unequal in Size, tho' fo exact in Likenefs, be Male and Female of the fame Species, I leave to the Judgment of the Curious. I find in *Willoughby* a very brief Account of a Bird, which I take to be this, it is *Bontius's Indian Stare*, *P.* 196 *Tab.* 38. For Whiftling, Singing and Talking, it is accounted in the firft Rank, expreffing Words with an Accent nearer Human than *Parrots* or any other Birds ufually taught to talk. They are faid to come from the Ifland *Borneo*, and 'tis likely they came from thence and the adjacent Parts. They are brought to us by the *India* Company's Ships. See Mr. *Albin's* Figure, in his *Hiftory of Birds, Vol. 2. Plate* 38

The

The SOLITARY SPARROW.

FOR Bignefs, Shape of Body, and Proportion of Parts, it is like the *Black-Bird*; the Figure reprefents the Bird of its natural Size. The Bill is ftraight, the upper Mandible bending a little downwards at the Point, of a black Colour above and beneath; the Infide and Corners of the Mouth of a redifh Yellow-colour; the Eye is of a dark Hazel-colour; the Eye-lids all round, of a yellow Colour; the Feathers of the whole Bird, except the Quills and Tail, are of a full Blue, darker on the Back, and lighter on the Breaft; the Feathers on the Breaft and Belly being bared acrofs or fringed with a lighter Colour; the Quills and Tail-feathers are of dusky Brown or Black, yet have they on their outer Webs fomething of Blue; fome of the firft Row of Wing Coverts, next the Belly, are tip'd with White; the Legs and Feet are Black; it hath black Claws.

This Bird is defcrib'd by *Willoughby*, P. 191. but there being no good Figure of it, I thought it might be acceptable to the Curious. They are fam'd for the Sweetnefs of their Singing. My Defcription differs a little from that in *Willoughby*; but I always choofe to defcribe from Nature itfelf, before I confult the Defcriptions of others. The Hen is defcrib'd, together with the Cock, in the above Page of *Willoughby*. I drew and defcrib'd this from the live Bird at Sir *Charles Wager*'s. They are faid to be found in the mountainous Parts of *Italy*, and breed in Rocks and old ruin'd Towers; but I have reafon to believe they are fcatter'd all over *Europe*, efpecially in the Southern Parts, fince I have feen fome of them that were fhot at *Gibraltar*, and fent dry'd to *London*.

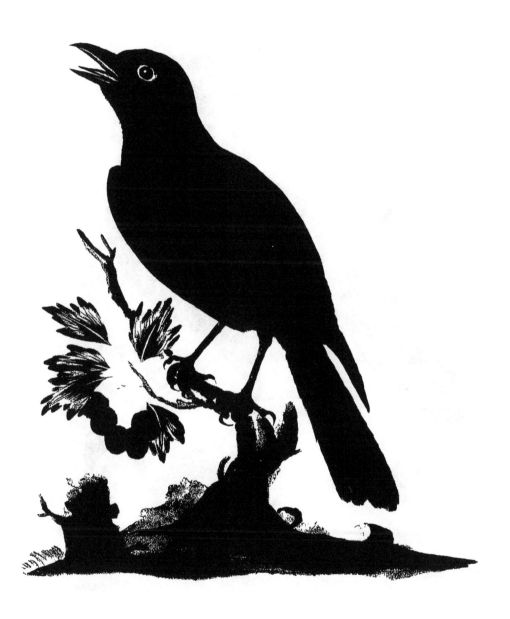

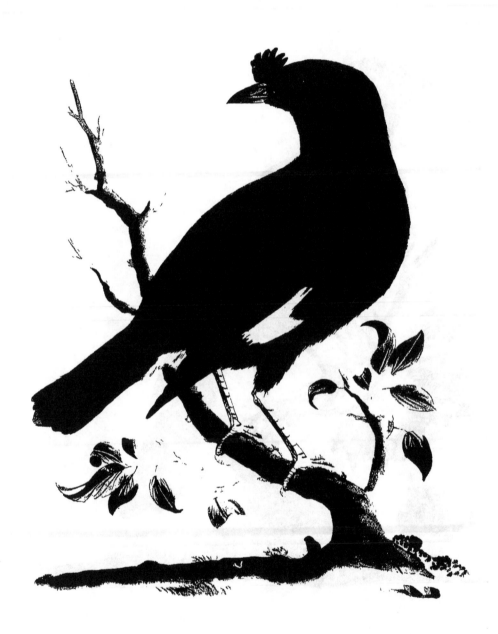

The CHINESE STARLING *or* BLACK-BIRD.

THIS Bird is call'd by our Sailors, who bring it from *China*, a *Martin*; but it being not of Kin to that Genus, I have taken the Liberty to change its Name, it being nearer of Kin to the *Starling*, than to any other *European* Bird; tho' it comes nearer to the *Minor* before defcrib'd, and is about the Bignefs of the leffer Sort of *Minor*; the Bill is pretty thick towards the Head, ftraight, grows gradually more flender, and ends in a Point, of a yellow Colour; yet the lower Mandible, towards the Head, inclines more to Red; the Noftrils are low on each Side, pretty near the Slit of the Mouth; the Eye is of a fine Gold or Orange-colour; it hath on the Forehead, juft at the Bafis of the Bill, a remarkable Tuft of Feathers, which it can erect at Pleafure in form of a Creft; the Crown of the Head is flat; the Head, Neck, whole Body, Wings and Tail, are of a black Colour, not gloffy and fhining with fplendid Colours, as in the *Minor*, nor quite fo dark as our common *Black-Bird*, but feems to incline a little to a dirty Blue; the Bottoms of fome of the firft Quills, next the Belly, are White, which form a white Spot in each Wing; tho' the Tail is Black, yet the fide Feathers are tip'd with White; the Legs and Feet are of a dull Yellow; the Claws of a light Colour.

This Bird being newly dead, the Iris of the Eye retaining its Luftre, was given to me by a Gentleman who brought it from *China*. I have fince feen fome of them alive in Bird-Merchants Hands, from whom I drew out Lines to improve my firft Draught. They are brought to us with much Difficulty, many dying for one that efcapes in the Voyage. They take to Whiftling and Talking pretty well. This Plate reprefents the natural Bignefs of the Bird. We fee it frequently drawn in Pictures brought to us from *China*; but no Natural Hiftorian, that I know of, hath given us any Draught or Defcription of it.

The Rose *or* Carnation-colour'd Ouzel *of* Aldrov. *Lib.* 16. *Cap.* 15.

THE Print here reprefents the Bird of its natural Bignefs; it is fhap'd pretty much like a *Starling*, tho' the Tail is fomething longer, yet not fo long as the *Black-Bird's*; it hath on its Head a Creft, here drawn as it appeared in the dead Bird preferv'd dry, which Creft erected in the living Bird muft, doubtlefs, appear very beautiful: The Bill is of a middling Length and Thicknefs, bowed a little downward and ending in a Point; the Point is of a black or dusky Colour, which gradually changes into a dirty Flefh-colour towards the Head; the Angles of the Mouth are pretty deep, reaching almoft under the Eyes; the whole Head, Neck, Wings and Tail, are Black, with a bright fhining Glofs of Blue, Purple and Green, changing Colour as it is differently turned to the Light; the Covert-feathers within-fide of the Wings are Black, with dirty white Edges; the Quills within-fide are of a dirty, blackifh Brown; the Breaft, Belly, Back, Rump, and leffer Coverts of the Wings, are of a Rofe or Bloffom-colour, feeming to be a Mixture of lighter and darker Parts; there are fprinkled on the Belly, Coverts of the Wings, and Rump, a few black Spots; the Thighs, lower Belly, and Coverts under the Tail, are of a dusky dull Black; the Legs and Feet are made after the ufual form, the outer and middle Toe join'd a little way; both Legs and Feet are of a dirty Orange-colour; the Claws Black.

I take this Bird to be a Cock, becaufe *Willoughby's* Defcription, *P.* 194. tranflated from *Aldrovandus*, fays the Hen hath not fo bright a Black as the Cock; it is faid to frequent Dung-heaps. *Willoughby's* Defcription feems to be too brief, therefore I choofe ftrictly to defcribe this Bird from Nature, having the Advantage of feeing it, which Mr. *Willoughby* had not: But whoever will take the trouble to compare this Defcription with that of *Aldrovandus*, I believe will agree with me that this muft be the fame Bird he has defcrib'd. You may fee this Bird very perfect, curioufly ftuffed and fet on a Perch at *Salter's* Coffee-houfe in *Chelfea*, where I had Liberty to draw it. Tho' this Bird is not a Native of *England*, yet it was fhot at *Norwood*, near *London*; for it often happens that Birds, not Natives of our Ifland, are, through Storms or other accidental Caufes unknown to us, brought over hither. The *Upupa* or *Hoopoe*, being alfo a foreign Bird, was fhot at *Norwood*, and is likewife preferv'd at *Salter's* Coffee-houfe with this.

The

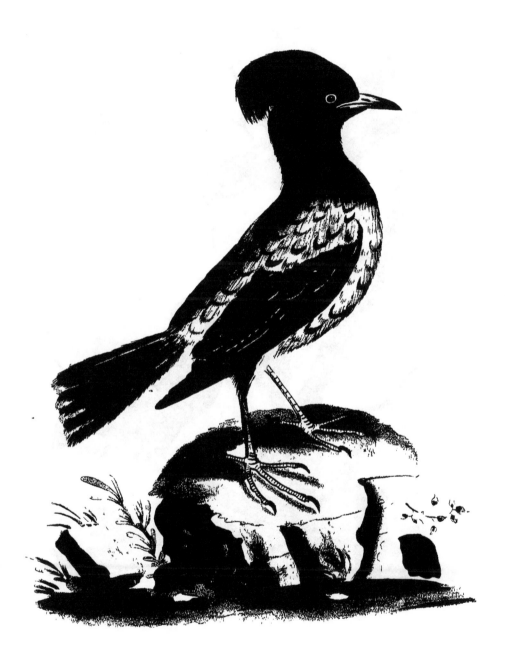

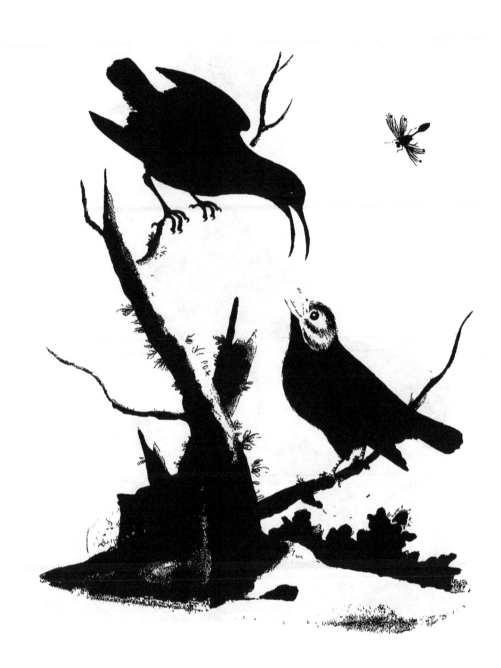

The BLUE CREEPER.

THE Figure shews the natural Bigness of this Bird. It hath a small Head, and a short Tail, the Bill agreeing in Shape with the *Certhia* or *Creeper*. I have given it that Name, tho' the Bill is a little longer, it being about an Inch long, slender, and bowed downward, of a blackish Colour; at the Base of the upper Mandible the Feathers are Black, which join with a black Line drawn from the Corners of the Mouth to the Eyes, under the Bill also is a black Mark, drawn a pretty way down the Throat, as in the *Cock Sparrow*, the whole Head and Body is of a fine deep Blue; the lesser Covert-feathers of the Wings are also Blue; the. prime Feathers, and the Row next above them, are Black, the Tail is short, very little exceeding the Length of the Wings, of a black Colour; the Legs, Feet, and Claws, are of a light yellow Brown.

♔ ♔

The GOLDEN-HEADED BLACK TIT-MOUSE.

THERE is no Genus of *European* Birds to which I can liken this Bird · It is pretty big-headed, round-body'd, short-tail'd and leg'd, it hath the Feet form'd directly as in the *King-fisher*, and wanteth only a long Bill to make it a perfect *King-fisher* I believe by its Feet and short Legs, it is of that Tribe, and may perhaps live and feed on Insects in Cane Swamps, as the *King-fisher* does on Fish, on the Borders of Rivers, but this is Conjecture   This Figure shews the Bird of its natural Size.   I have seen *Dutch* Drawings of these Birds, entitled, *Manakins*, which is a Name the *Hollanders* give to some *European* Birds also, it hath a short Bill, not thick or very slender, but shap'd like the Bills of *Tit-mice*, of a white Colour, the Crown, hinder Part of the Head and under the Eyes, are of a bright Orange or Golden-colour; the Throat, whole Body, Wings and Tail, are Black, yet shining with a blue or purplish Gloss when exposed to a good Light, the Feathers covering each Knee are of an Orange-colour, the Legs very short, the Toes as in *King-fishers*, with small Claws, the Legs, Feet, and Claws, are all of a Flesh-colour.

These two curious Birds, above describ'd, were lent me by his Grace the Duke of *Richmond*.   They are neatly set up, with many others, in Glass-Cases   they were sent to the Duke from *Holland*, who told me they came from *Surinam*, a *Dutch* Settlement on the Continent of *South America*, which lies in a very warm Latitude.   I have called it a *Tit-mouse*, because it hath a Bill like that Tribe of Birds, and is of the same Size, but I do not think it a Species belonging to that Genus.   I have seen Drawings of both these Birds in the Collections of the Curious, but no Figures of them have been publish'd with Descriptions, that I know of.

G

The

The RED-BELLY'D BLUE-BIRD.

THIS Plate ſhews the Bird of the bigneſs of Life; it is of that Tribe which *Willoughby* has call'd *Slender-bill'd Birds*, whoſe Tails are all of one Colour, of which Number is the *Nightingale*, *Robin Red-breaſt*, *Redſtart*, and many other *Engliſh* Small Birds; it hath a ſlender ſharp-pointed Bill, of a middling Length, of a dark Lead-colour; the Head, Neck, Breaſt, Wings, Tail, and upper Part of the Back, are of a purpliſh blue Colour, partly very bright, partly obſcure; the Sides of the Head, the Breaſt, and the Coverts of the Wings, are the brighter Parts; the upper Part of the Neck and Back, of a dull dirty Blue, partaking a little of Green; from the under Part of the Bill, a little way down the Throat, is of a dirty Blue or dark Colour; the Quills and Tail-feathers are of a black or dusky Colour, the Edges of the Feathers being Blue; the lower Part of the Back is of a light Colour, with a faint Mixture of Roſe; the Covert-feathers of the Tail of a fine blue purple Colour; the Thighs, lower Belly, and Coverts under the Tail, are of a dirty rediſh Orange-colour; the Legs, Feet, and Claws, of a dark Lead-colour.

I was favour'd with a Draught of this Bird by his Grace the Duke of *Richmond*: It was brought from *Surinam*. I believe this Bird hath not before been deſcrib'd.

The SCARLET LOCUST.

THE Figure preſents you the natural Bigneſs of this Inſect: The Head and Horns are of a dull Red; the Scale or Shell, which covers the middle of the Body, of a bright Red, and rough like Sha-green; the Wings of a dull Red; the hinder Part was compoſed of black and ſcarlet Rings quite round; the under Side of the middle of the Body of a dirty Red; the Legs of a bright Scarlet, except the Joints, which were black.

This Inſect came accidentally alive from the *Weſt Indies* in a Basket of Pine-Apples. It was given me by Dr. *R. M. Maſſey*: It fed on Vine-Leaves, and lived a whole Summer in *England*.

The

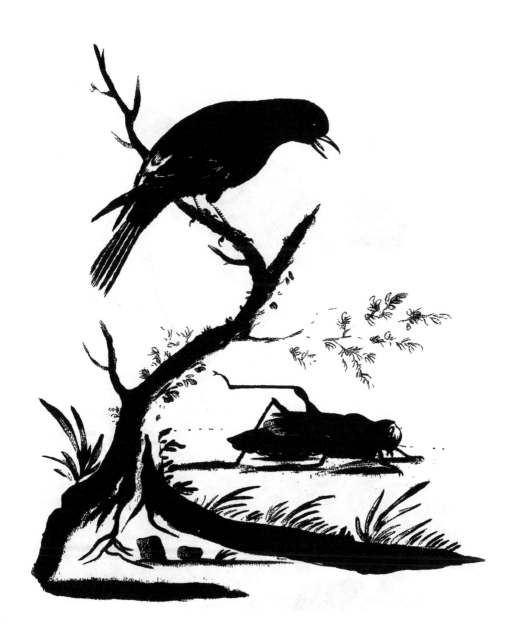

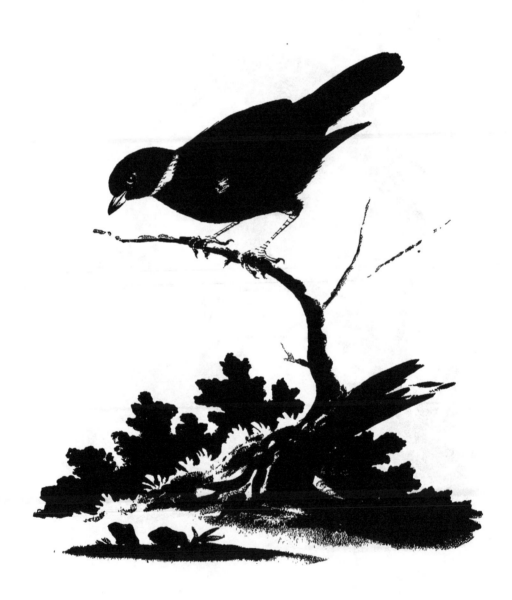

The RED-HEADED GREEN-FINCH.

THIS is of the Number of very beautiful Birds; it is here figur'd
of the bignefs of Life: I take it rather to be of the thick and
hard-bill'd Kind, than of flender-bill'd Birds, who live moftly on Infects,
yet the Bill is not fo big in Proportion as in moft fmall Birds, call'd *Hard-
bill'd Birds*; but many *American* Birds differ fo much in little Circum-
ftances, that one cannot eafily conclude what *European* Birds to range
them with: The Bill is of a light brownifh or Horn-colour; its Shape is
very well exprefs'd in the Figure; the Head is of a red Colour, not bright
Scarlet, but fomething dull, and inclining to a high-colour'd Orange;
round the Neck is a yellow Ring, which points upwards a little under the
Bill; the Neck, Back, Wings and Tail, are of a fine Parrot-green; the
greater Quills towards their Pips, are dusky; on the upper Part of the
Wing near the Joint or Bend, is a roundifh yellow Spot, near half an
Inch in Breadth; the Breaft and Belly, as low as the Thighs, are of a
pleafant light blue Colour; the upper Part of the Thighs, lower Belly,
and under the Tail, are Green; part of the Thighs next the Legs are
Yellow; the Legs, Feet, and Claws, of a light brown Colour.

This Bird is in the Duke of *Richmond*'s Cabinet; it came from *Surinam.* Where my Subjects have been Birds out of Spirits, or otherwife
preferv'd, I have made no mention of the Colour of their Eyes, not
knowing what Colour they have been of; though a Brother Author that
has lately publifhed fome hundreds of Birds, was not pleafed to do fo, for he
has given Irides of very beautiful and fhining Colours, both in Defcription and Colouring, to many Birds which he never faw alive, or newly
dead, or any Perfon who could inform him. Mr. *Dandridge* in *More-
fields* is poffefs'd of many of the Birds, from which his Defcriptions were
taken, who has told me, that he himfelf never knew what Colour the
Eyes of thefe Birds were of, fo could not pretend to tell it to another. I cannot find that the above-defcrib'd Bird has been before taken
notice of by any one.

The BLUE RED-BREAST.

THIS Bird feems to be of that Tribe or Family of flender-bill'd Birds who feed on Infects: The Print gives its natural Size, or if there be any Difference, the Bird is rather bigger than the Figure, if I, contrary to Cuftom, may be allow'd to point out my own Miftakes: It is fhap'd like a *Redftart*; the Bill is fharp-pointed, flender, of a moderate Length and dusky Colour; the whole upper Side, Head, Neck, Back, Wings and Tail, are of a fine full blue Colour, except the Ends of the greater Quills, which are Black with brown Tips; the whole under Side, from the Bill to the Covert-feathers under the Tail, is of a redifh Colour; juft under the Bill, White, or very light Ruffet; on the Breaft the Colour gradually heightens to a full Orange, or the Colour of a *Robin*'s Breaft; towards the Belly the Colour dies again into a faint Red, and fo continues to the Covert-feathers of the Tail; the Thighs are of the fame faint or light Red; the Legs and Feet, which are form'd and ftand after the ufual manner, are of a brown Colour; it hath dusky Claws.

I had this Bird of Mr. *Peter Colinfon*, who, I think, told me it came from *Bermudas*. Mr. *Catesby* has, in his Hiftory of *Carolina*, *Vol* 1. *p.* 47. defcrib'd and figur'd a Bird nearly refembling this, which he calls fimply the *Blue-Bird*; but as this differs fomething from his Bird, I thought it would not be amifs to figure and defcribe it under the above Name. The only difference between this Bird and his, is, that the red Colour in mine was continued quite to the Bill; his was Blue on the under Side of the Neck, from the Bill to the beginning of the Breaft, and by his Defcription mine feems to be of a brighter Red on the Breaft, yet I believe them to be the fame or near of Kin. I fhould not have prefumed to re-publifh any thing that was directly the fame with what has been publifhed by Mr. *Catesby*, becaufe I know myfelf not capable to add any Amendments to what he has done. Mr. *Catesby* has call'd his Bird *Rubecula Americana*, which is a proper Name enough, fince both his Bird and mine are certainly of that Genus, of which the *Robin Red-breaft* is a Species.

The

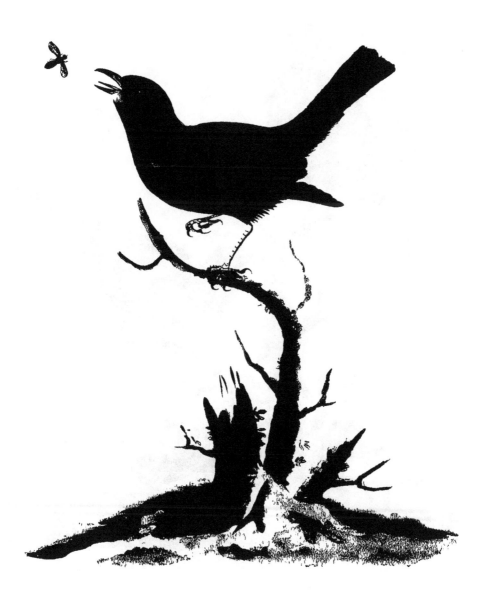

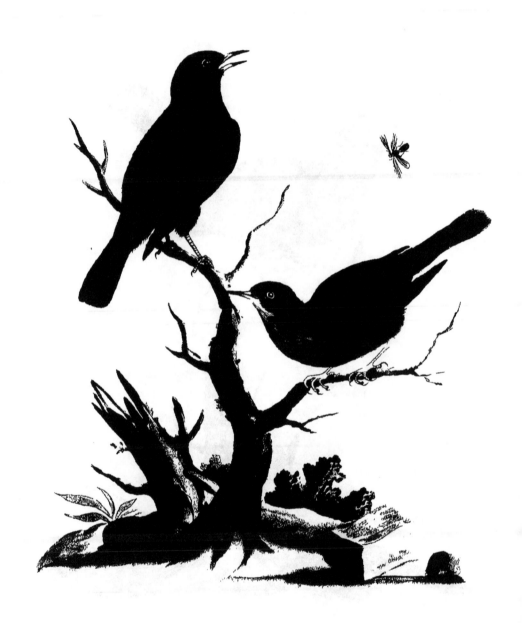

The GREEN BLACK-CAP FLY-CATCHER.

THIS Bird is figur'd of its natural Bigness; for shape of Body it's like a *Robin Red-breast*; the Bill is slender, of a middling Length, bowed downward a very little towards the Point, which is sharp, of a dusky or Horn-colour above, the lower Mandible lighter, both a little Yellow next the Head; the Crown, Sides, and hinder Parts of the Head, are cover'd as it were with a Cap of black Feathers, having a Point or Corner under each Eye; the Eyes are placed on each Side the Head in the middle of the black Part; the Throat, quite to the Bill, and the whole remaining Part of the Bird, is of an equal blue-green Colour; the Quills are something darker than the other Parts, especially the greater or outer Quills, which lose their Greenness by degrees, and become blackish at their Tips; the Legs and Feet, which conform to the usual Shape, in small Birds, are of a dark Lead-colour.

The BLUE-HEADED GREEN FLY-CATCHER.

THIS Bird, in Figure and Magnitude, is equal to the above-describ'd, or if there be any Difference on comparing the Birds themselves, I thought this rather the least; the Shape of the Bill is the same with the above; it is of a light Ash-colour or White, in the upper Part lightest at the Base, the lower Mandible is of a darker Ash-colour; the Top and Sides of the Head are of a light Blue-colour; the Throat, just under the Bill, is White, for a small Space; the Neck, whole Body, and Tail, are of a very yellowish Green; the Wing on the Shoulder, or Part next the Head, hath a roundish Spot of Blue; the Covert-feathers and Quills, except the Greater, are Yellow-green, like the Body, the greater Quills are of a dark Brown, or black Colour; the under Side of the Tail is dusky; the Legs and Feet of a faint yellow Colour.

Thefe two Birds are preserved in the Cabinet of his Grace the Duke of *Richmond*, they are Natives of *Surinam*. They being so like in Shape and Colour, I am inclined to believe them Male and Female of the same Species; but it is hard to determine any thing absolutely, unless one had been in the Country, where they are Natives, and made particular Observations of them. These Birds may be ranged with slender-bill'd Small Birds, whose Tails are all of one Colour. I believe these Birds have not before been figur'd or describ'd.

H

The

The little BROWN and WHITE CREEPER.

THIS Bird I have call'd the *Creeper*, from the Conformity of all its Parts with the *European Certhia*, tho' it is not above half the Bigness, nor hath it the beautiful Spots and Marks which our *Creeper* hath, yet the general Colour, Shape of the Body and Bill, are the same; it is here represented of its natural Bigness; the Bill is about three-fourths of an Inch long, of a middling Thickness at its Base, bowed downwards, ending in a sharp Point, of a dark brown Colour; the upper Sides of the Head, Neck, Back and Wings, are of a brown inclining to Copper-colour; the whole under Side, from Bill to Tail, is White; it hath a Bar of dark Brown, passing from the Corners of the Mouth to the Eyes, from the Sides of the upper Mandible of the Bill passes white Lines above the Eyes, on each Side the Covert-feathers, within-side the Wings are White; the greater Quills are of a darker Brown than the rest of the Body, the Edges of the Feathers being something light, the Tail is dark Brown or Black, the outermost Feathers on each Side, having white Tips; the Legs, Feet, and Claws, Brown.

This Bird preserv'd in Spirits, was lent me by Dr. *Cromwell Mortimer*; he brought it from *Holland*, and was informed it came from the *East Indies*. I took it out of the Spirits in order to draw it. The Glass which contain'd it was titled with a *Dutch* Name, which in *English* signifies the *Honey Thief*. I believe this Bird hath not been till now either figur'd or describ'd.

I Do not pretend to have any Skill in the Description of Insects, not having at all study'd them; nor do I know the Terms by which their Parts are distinguished: But they being no Part of my Design, I have added them only as Decorations to fill up some void Spaces in the Plates where the Birds were small; so that if my Descriptions are obscure, I hope the Justness of the Figures will help to clear them. The Head and Body of this Fly is Black on the upper Side, the upper Wing mostly Black, having two redish Spots near the Body, then a broad, and after it a narrow brown Mark; toward the Ends are two Eyes of Blue, surrounded with Red, and across each End a Mark like Beads of a light Brown, under the greater Eyes of Blue, toward the lower Wing, is a Spot of Blue; the lower Wings are blue in the Middle, black at their Roots, border'd with Stripes of Black and light Brown, having in each Wing two pretty large Eyes, blue in the Middle, red without that, and black Rings without the Red. On the under Side of the Fly the Head is redish, the Body light Brown; the upper Wing barred across with Orange-colour and Black, having a pretty large Eye of Black, encompass'd by Orange, the under Wing of a dark purplish Colour, with Spots and transverse Lines of Black.

This Fly, with many others, were presented me by Capt. *Isaac Worth*, now in the *India* Company's Service. It came from *China*.

The

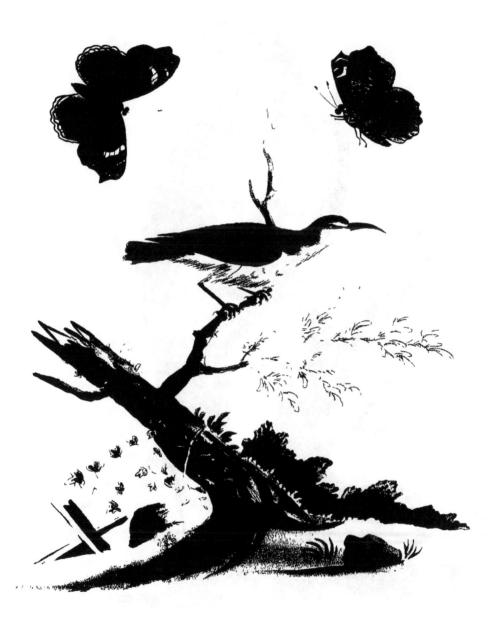

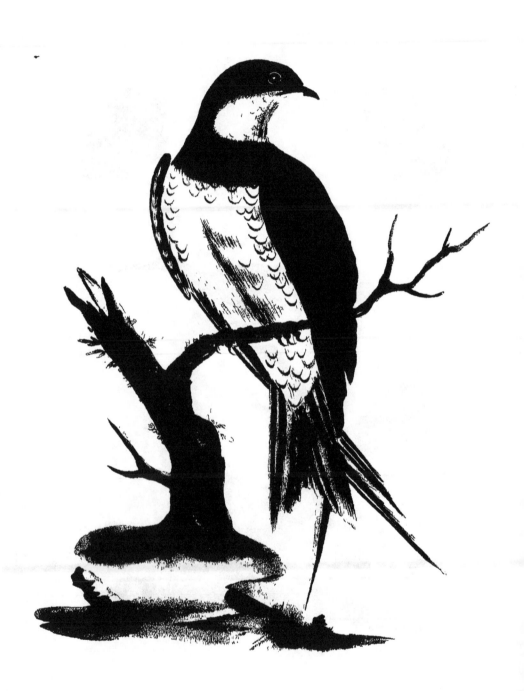

The Greateſt MARTIN *or* SWIFT.

THIS Bird in Shape is like the common *Black Martin* or *Swift*, but I believe twice the Bigneſs; the Head ſomething flat, and pretty broad, the Bill ſmall, the Slit of the Mouth deep, reaching under the Eyes, the Neck ſhort, the Wings very long, the Tail of a moderate Length. This Plate ſhews the Bird of its natural Bigneſs, or rather leſs, if it differs from the Truth, the Bird being dry'd with the Body remaining in the Skin, the Bill is black, a little hooked at the Point, the upper Side of the Head, Neck, Back, Wings, and Tail, are of a dirty brown Colour; the Back and Rump however, are ſomething lighter, tho' of the ſame brown Colour, the outer or firſt Quills are of a darker Brown than the other Parts, which happens in moſt Birds; the inſide of the Quills, and under-ſide of the Tail, are of a fainter Brown inclining to Aſh-colour, from the Bill, downward, the Throat is white, on the lower Part of the Neck it hath a Bar of Brown ſpotted with Black, in form of a Collar, the Breaſt and Belly are white, the Thighs, lower Belly, and Covert-feathers under the Tail, are of a light Brown, or rather dirty White; the Sides of the Breaſt and Belly, near the Wings, are mixed a little with brown Marks, the Edges of ſome of the Feathers being Brown; the Legs are ſhort, and cover'd with fine downy Feathers of a light Colour; the Toes, four in Number, ſeem'd to ſtand all forward, of a black Colour, as are the Claws. This Bird ſo nearly reſembles the *Leſſer Martin*, call'd the *Sand* or *Bank Martin*, that the Deſcription of the one might almoſt ſerve for the other, ſave that this is as large as a *Black-Bird*, or very near it, and that very little bigger than a *Wren*

I had this Bird of Mr. *Catesby*, who has obliged me with many new and curious Birds to draw after. It was ſhot on the Rocks of *Gibraltar*, by a Brother of Mr. *Catesby*'s, who reſided ſome time there. *Gibraltar* being ſo near to *Africa*, 'tis probable the Birds of Paſſage may paſs in Flocks from *Europe* to *Barbary*, and from thence to *Europe* at certain Seaſons. It would be worthy the Obſervation of *Engliſh* Gentlemen who reſide there, to take particular Notice if there be any ſuch Paſſages there, and what Birds they are that paſs, and at what Seaſons they go *Southward*, and at what Times they return *Northward*, which might give ſome Light to the paſſing of Birds, which at preſent we know very little of. It is hardly to be thought that Land Birds ſhould chooſe wide Seas to paſs over, when ſo ſhort a Cut is to be found.

The BLUE-THROAT REDSTART.

THIS Bird is bigger than the common *Redstart*; it's of the Size here exprefs'd; for Shape, like other fmall Birds of this Kind. I have feen a Drawing of it from *Holland* or *Germany*, which was named *Bláu-kehle*, which is *Blue-throat*, and it being fo near of Kin to the *Redstart*, I have given it the above Name. The Bill is ftraight, moderately long and flender, of a black Colour; the upper-fide of the Head, Neck, Back and Wings, is of a dark dirty Brown, the Edges of the Feathers being lighter; above the Eye paffes a Line of dirty Orange-colour; from the Corner of the Mouth under the Eye, paffes another Line of the fame Colour; beneath this paffes a narrow Line of faint Blue; the Throat, from the Bill downward, is white; on the lower Part of the Neck is a Spot of Blue like a Half-moon, the Corners pointing upwards; the beginning of the Breaft, for a fmall Space, is of an Orange-colour, narrower in the Middle, reaching a little farther down on the Sides; the remainder of the Breaft, Belly, Thighs, and Covert-feathers under the Tail is white; the two middle Feathers of the Tail are dark Brown, the other Feathers on each Side are Orange-colour with blackifh Tips half an Inch deep; the Covert-feathers on the upper Side of the Tail are of a dirty Orange-colour; the Legs, Feet, and Claws are brown.

I had this Bird of Mr. *Catesby*; it was fent from *Gibraltar* to him.

The

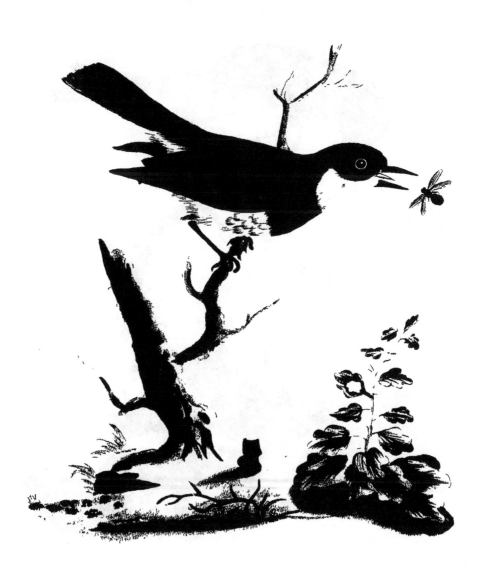

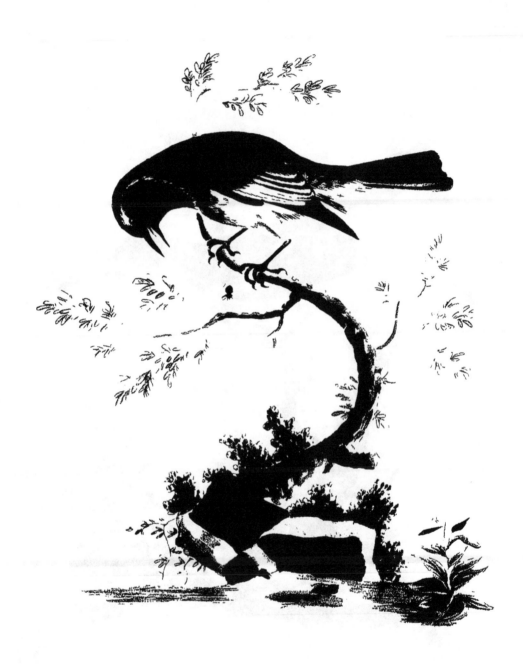

The GREY REDSTART.

THE Figure here gives you the natural Size of the Bird; it is near
the Size and Shape of the common *Redftart*; the Bill is flender,
ftraight, of a moderate Length, and dark brown Colour; the Forehead,
for a little Space above the Bill, and the Sides of the Head and Throat are
black; on the fore-part of the Head behind the Black, is a narrow Space
of White, which extends itfelf backward above the Eyes on each Side;
the Top of the Head, Neck, Back, Breaft and Covert-feathers of the
Wings, are of a bluifh Grey or Afh-colour; the Quill-feathers are a
little more inclining to Brown; the outer Webs of the middlemoft
Quills are White, except juft at the Tips, which Whitenefs forms a
longifh white Spot on the Wing when the Feathers are clofed; the Rump
and Covert-feathers of the Tail, both above and beneath, are of a bright
Orange-colour; the two middle Feathers of the Tail are Brown, the
Feathers next them Orange-colour, having fmall brown Tips; the outer-
moft Feathers on each Side wholly Orange-colour; the lower Belly and
Thighs of a white Colour; the Legs, Feet and Claws of a dusky or
brownifh Colour.

I had this Bird of Mr. *Catesby*, it was fent to him from *Gibraltar*
in *Old Spain*. I believe this Bird hath not yet been figur'd or defcrib'd.

I

The

The *Cock* COLD FINCH.

THIS is the *Baccafigo* or *Ficedula Tertia* of *Aldrovand* The Bird is of the Shape and Bigness of the uppermost Figure in the Plate; the Bill is slender, straight, and of a black Colour, the Eye is Hazel-colour'd; on the Forehead, a little above the Bill, is a white Spot, the Crown, Sides of the Head, upper-part of the Neck and Back, are Black; the Rump and Coverts of the Tail are black and white mixed; the whole under-side is pure White; the Covert-feathers of the Wings are Brown, as are the outermost Quills; the inner Quills next the Body, have their exterior Webs White, the interior Black; the Tips of the Covert-feathers next above the Quills, are White; which, together with the White on the Quills, form a large white Spot, the Edges of the outer Quills are of a lighter Brown than the other Parts of the Feathers; the middle Part of the Tail is Black, but the outermost Feathers on each Side have the outer Shafts White, the next Feathers to them are White only toward their Bottoms; the Legs, Feet, and Claws, are Black.

The *Hen* COLD FINCH.

THE Bill, Eyes, Legs, Feet, and whole under-side of the Body, agree with that above; the Top of the Head, Neck, Back, Rump, and lesser Coverts of the Wings, are of a dirty greenish Brown; the greater Quills are Brown; the lesser, or those next the Back, have the outer Webs yellowish White, the inner Dusky, the first Row of Coverts above the Quills is Black, with white Tips; which, with the White in the Quills, make a white Spot in the Wing; the Sides under the Wings, and the Covert-feathers within-side of the Wings in both Birds are White; the middle Feathers of the Tail are Dusky, the outer edg'd with White. I take this to be the Hen of the Bird above describ'd, tho' *Willoughby*'s Description mentions the Testicles, which might proceed from this Cause, that the Cocks and Hens, in some Birds, in their first Feathers differ hardly at all, tho' when they have moulted, there is a great Difference as in these, the Head and Back in the one is Black, in the other a brownish Green or Olive, in other things they agree pretty well.

I could find no Figures of these scarce Birds, tho' we have Descriptions, therefore I thought they might be acceptable to the Curious They are something otherwise described in *Willoughby* than I have done them, but I do not choose to repeat the Descriptions of others, (though better than mine) when I have Nature before me. These Birds were lent me by *Taylor White*, Esq, who procur'd them from the *Peak* in *Derbyshire*

This last Bird is describ'd in *Willoughby*, *p.* 236. by the Name of *Cold Finch*, but as his Description differs something from mine I suspect that his was taken from the Cock-Bird, before it had moulted its first Feathers. These Birds were shot together

The

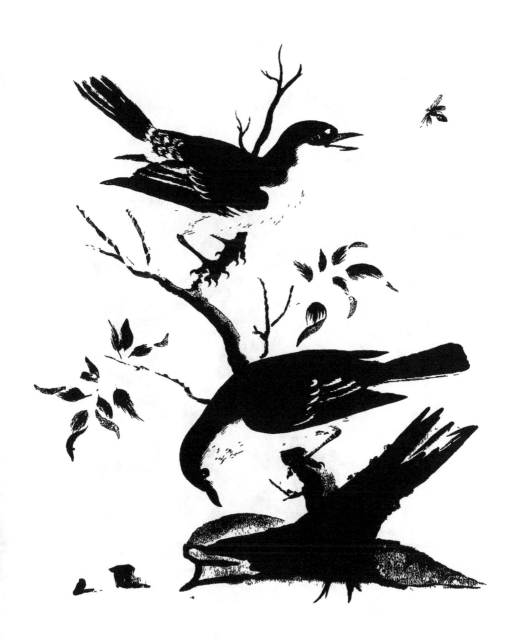

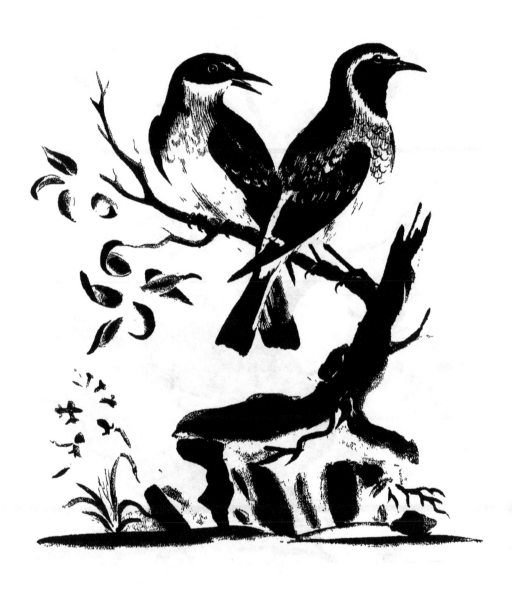

The RED *or* RUSSET-COLOUR'D WHEAT-EAR.

THESE Birds feem'd to be about the Bignefs of *Sparrows*; I have figur'd them of the natural Bignefs as near as I could. The Cock, which I fuppofe to be that with the black Throat, has a ftraight, flender, black or dark Lead-colour'd Bill; a little Space at the Bafe of the upper Mandible, the Cheeks, under the Eyes and Throat, from the Bill about an Inch downwards, are Black; there paffes round this black Space, a whitifh Line, broader on the Forehead and above the Eyes, narrower downwards on the Throat; the Top of the Head, Neck, Back and Breaft, are of a dirty faint Orange-colour, inclining to Buff, deeper on the Back, fainter on the Breaft; the lower Part of the Back is fpotted with femi-lunar Spots of Black; the Rump, lower Part of the Belly, Thighs, and Covert-feathers under the Tail are White; the whole Wing Black or very dark dusky Brown; the Tips and Edges of the Feathers next above the Quills, and of fome of the Quills next the Back, are of a lightifh Brown; the Legs, Feet, and Claws, dark Brown or Black; the middle Feathers of the Tail are black or dusky, the fide Feathers are white with black Tips, of a fmall Depth.

THE other Bird, which I believe to be the Hen of the above-defcrib'd, hath a little Black at the Root of the upper Part of the Bill, which paffes from the Corners of the Bill through the Eyes, and becomes pretty broad behind the Eyes; the Chin, beneath the Bill, is White; the whole Body, Wings, Tail, and Legs, agree with the above-defcrib'd; this Bird being very near of Kin to the *Oenanthe* or *Wheat Ear*, defcrib'd in *Willoughby*, *p.* 233. I knew not what Name to give it better than the above, with the Diftinction join'd to it.

Thefe Birds, which agree with no Figures or Defcriptions I can find, came from *Gibraltar*, where they were fhot by a Gentleman refiding there, who fent them to Mr. *Catesby* in *London*, who favour'd me with a Sight of them, from which I made thefe Draughts and Defcriptions.

The

The LONG-TAIL'D RED HUMING-BIRD.

THIS Bird is one of the largeſt of the Kind I have met with, as well as the moſt beautiful; it is here fignr'd of its natural Bigneſs: I believe it had loſt one of the long Feathers of the Tail, becauſe I never obſerv'd any Bird to have an odd or ſingle Feather in its Tail, that had not its like or fellow. The Bill of this Bird is long, ſlender, and bowed down toward the Point, of a black Colour; the Head, and upper Part of the Neck are Black, with a ſhining Luſtre; the Throat is of the moſt ſplendid Colour one can conceive, being Green ſhining with the Luſtre of poliſh'd Gold; below this Green is a black ſemi-lunar Line parting it from the Breaſt, which is of a Roſe-colour; the Back and Covert-feathers of the Wings are Red, but more inclining to Orange than the Breaſt; the Quills and Row of Coverts next above them, are of a dull Purple-colour; the Tail hath two long Feathers in the middle, of the ſame Purple with the Wings; the Side-feathers of the Tail are rediſh Orange like the Back, the lower Part of the Back, Rump, and Coverts of the Tail, are of a fine Green-colour; the Legs and Feet are Black; it hath very ſhort Legs, and four Toes, ſtanding three forward and one backward, as all of this Kind have.

The Little BROWN HUMING-BIRD.

THIS is one of the leaſt of the *Huming-Bird* Kind I have met with, being no bigger than the upper Figure in this Plate repreſents it; the Bill is long, ſlender, a little bowed or bent downward, the upper Mandible longer than the nether, of a dark or black Colour; the lower Mandible is Fleſh-colour'd toward the Head, black at the Point, the Top of the Head is dirty Brown, ſpotted with bright Brown, the Throat, Sides of the Head, all round the Neck, Breaſt and Belly, are of a bright Bay or dirty Orange-colour; under the Eye is a ſtroke of dark Brown or Black, and ſome dark Spots in the middle of the Breaſt, the Back, and upper Part of the Wings, are of a dirty brown Colour, intermixed with brighter yellowiſh Brown, the Quills and Tail-feathers, (except the middle Feathers, which are brown) are of a dirty Purple-colour; the Legs, Feet, and Claws, black.

I think this is the only Bird of this Genus that hath no Green nor ſhining Gold-like Luſtre mixed in its Feathers. Theſe Birds are preſerved in the Cabinet of his Grace the Duke of *Richmond*. They were brought from *Surinam*.

The

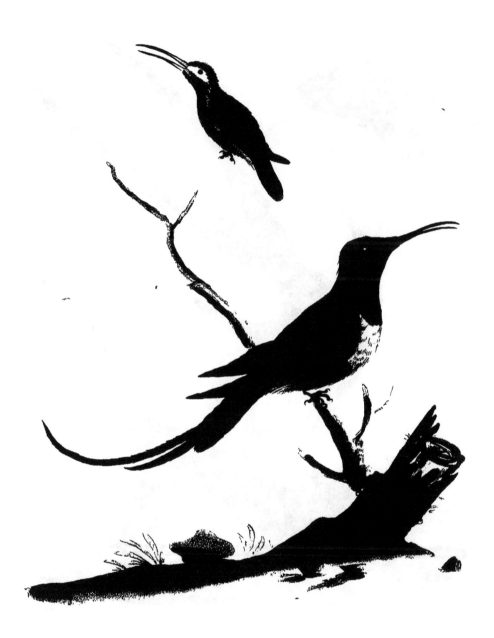

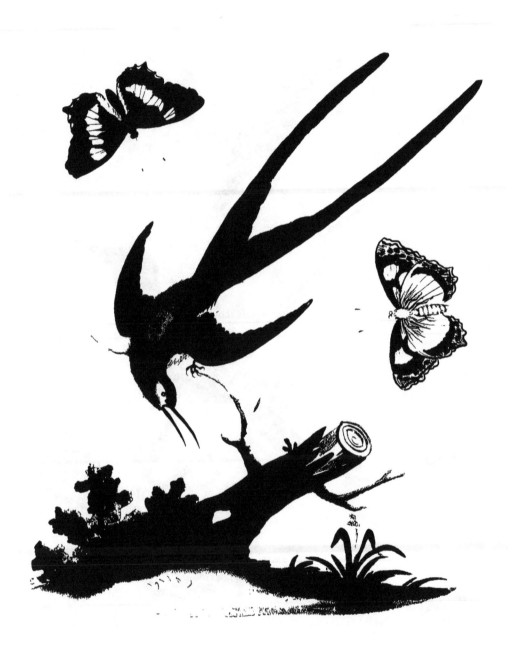

The LONG-TAIL'D GREEN HUMING BIRD.

THE Figure of this Bird is of the natural Bigneſs; it hath a very long and broad Tail, in proportion to the Body, the Feathers being very firm and ſtiff, not eaſily put in Diſorder; the Bill is ſlender, ſtraight, pretty long, and of a black Colour; the Crown of the Head is Blue, or elſe the Bird is moſtly Green; the Quills are of a dirty purpliſh Colour, except three Green ones next the Body; the Coverts of the Wings are Green; the lower Belly, and Coverts under the Tail, are White, the Thighs dusky; the Tail-feathers are of the moſt ſhining Beauty that can be imagined, appearing ſometimes of a ſhining Blue-colour, and upon a little turn will change Greeniſh, then again into a Colour mixed with a bright golden Splendor; the Feathers, all over the Body, have ſomething of a ſhining golden Luſtre, but nothing in compariſon with the Beauty of the Tail; the Legs, Feet, and Claws, are black.

This Bird was brought from *Jamaica* by Capt. *Chandler* at *Stepney*, of whom I procur'd leave to take a Drawing of it.

THE upper Side of this *Butter-Fly* is black, having in the upper Wings two white Spots in each; the lower Wings have each one large white Spot, and a ſmall round red Spot, beſides little faint white Marks between the Scolops of the Wings; the under Side of the Body is white; the lower Wings have each a large roundiſh white Spot, border'd on the upper Sides with Red, the Extremes of the Wings of a dirty Colour, ſpotted with Purple; within theſe purple Spots is a Bar of Black, with a Row of ſcarlet Spots in it; the upper Wings have three white Spots, that neareſt the Body border'd with a bent Bar of Red, the Spaces between the white Spots, Black, the Extremity of the Wing dusky, with purple Spots, and within them ſcarlet Spots on Black.

I was told by Mr. *William Goupey*, who lent me this *Fly*, that it came from the *Eaſt Indies*; but he could not tell from what particular Part.

K

The

The LONG-TAIL'D BLAK-CAP HUMING BIRD.

THIS Bird is engraved of its natural Bigneſs; it hath a longer Tail than the laſt deſcribed; the two long Feathers being of a looſe, ſoft Texture, eaſily ruffled and flowing with the leaſt Breath of Air; what is remarkable in the Tail is, that theſe two fine Feathers are the outermoſt but one on each Side, having a leſſer ſtiff Feather under them, as well as above, the better to ſupport them, which is ſingular. So far as my Obſervation reaches, all Birds, whoſe Tail-feathers differ in Length, have either the two middlemoſt or the two outermoſt the longeſt, as in the *Swallow* and *Magpye*, the Bill is thicker at the Baſis than in moſt of this Kind, pretty long, ending in a Point, a little bowed downward, of a yellow Colour, with a black Point; the Crown of the Head, and beginning of the Neck behind, is of a black Colour, with ſomething of a bluiſh Gloſs, the Throat, Breaſt, and Belly, are cover'd with Green Feathers, inclining to Blue, of a firm Subſtance, lying cloſe and regular like the Scales of Fiſhes, and of ſo fine a Surface, that they reflect the Light as doth burniſhed **Gold**; the Feathers on the Back are of a looſer Make, of a yellower Green, not having the bright Luſtre of the Breaſt, the Wings are of a browniſh Purple, having, in ſome Lights, a brighter bluiſh purple Caſt, the Ridge of the Wing from the Shoulder, a good way down, is white, the Tail is black or duſky, the Feathers increaſing in Length from the middle-moſt to the outermoſt ſave one, which is about five Times longer than any of the reſt, the Legs, Feet, and Claws, are black.

Mr. *P. Colinſon* obliged me with a Sight of this Bird I ſaw another that came with it, in the Repoſitory of the *Royal Society*, which differ'd only a little in Size from this. They were brought from *Jamaica*. I never could find above ten Feathers in the Tail of any Bird of this Genus.

The duſky *and* yellow Swallow-tail'd BUTTER-FLY.

THIS *Fly* was given me by Dr. *R. M. Maſſey*, who told me he had it from *Maryland*. The Ground of the Body and Wings are of a dirty dark Brown, barred and ſpotted (as the Print will direct better than the Deſcription) with Yellow, or rather Brimſtone-colour; all the Spots and Marks on the whole *Fly* being yellowiſh, except two Half-moon-like Spots neareſt the Point of the Tail, which are bright Red.

The

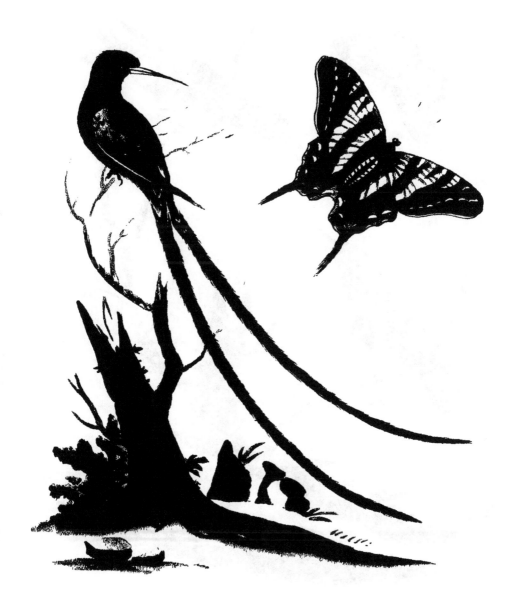

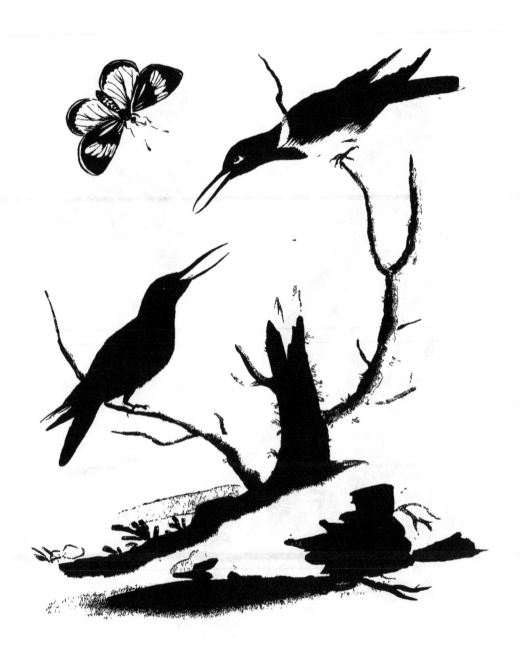

The WHITE-BELLY'D HUMING BIRD.

THIS Bird, and the Bird defcrib'd under it, are figur'd in the Plate, of their natural Bignefs, the Bill is pretty long, ftraight, and flender, the Points of the
upper and lower Mandibles a little bending towards each other, of a black Colour; the
whole Head and Neck, above and beneath, of a fine Blue, the Back, Rump, and
leffer Covert-feathers of the Wings of a fine Green, at the bottom of the Neck behind, is a white Mark, in the form of a Crefcent, the Horns pointing upwards, the
Belly is white, the Wings are Copper-colour, inclining to Purple; the middle Feathers
of the Tail are Green, the fide Feathers White, and fomething longer than the middle
Feathers, the Legs and Feet of a dark or blackifh Colour, the Colours in this Bird,
as in moft of this Kind, feem to be mixed with fine golden Threads, which make the
whole Bird appear very fplendid, when expofed to the Sun-beams.

The GREEN *and* BLUE HUMING BIRD.

AS this Bird was brought over with the other, and they agreeing in Shape, Size,
Form of the Bill and Feet, I have conjectur'd they may be Male and Female,
but I leave that to the Determination of the Curious, or future Difcovery, the Bill is
altogether like that above defcribed; the whole Head and Neck Green; the Breaft
and upper Part of the Back, Blue, the Thighs and lower Belly of a dirty brown
Colour, the leffer Covert-feathers of the Wings, the lower Part of the Back and
Rump Green; but the Rump is of an orient Caft, fhining with a golden Glofs, as do
the Colours on the Throat and Breaft, the Quills and firft Row of Coverts, are of a
dirty Copper-colour, a little inclining to Purple, the Tail of the fame purplifh Colour,
the Legs and Feet, Black
    Thefe Birds came together from *Surinam,* and are both preferved in the Cabinet of
his Grace the Duke of *Richmond.*

The Brown *and* White-fpotted BUTTER-FLY *from* China.

THE Print fhews its full Magnitude; the upper Wings are dark Brown, ftreaked
and fpotted with White; the extreme Borders, both of the upper and under
Wings, are White, the under Wings are White, except a Border of Brown near their
extreme Edges, plain outwards, and indented inwards; the Body is White, with black
Spots, the Head is Orange-colour, as is the Tail for three Joints or Rings from the
Tip

The

The BLACK-BELLY'D GREEN HUMING BIRD.

THESE Birds are figur'd of their natural Size; they are of the larger Sort of *Huming Birds*; the Bills in both are long, flender, and a little bent downward, not very fharp-pointed, of a black Colour; the Head, Neck, Back, and leffer Coverts of the Wings, in the upper Bird, are of a bluifh Green-colour; the fcapular Feathers, or thofe between the Back and Wings, have fomething of Red mixed with the Green; the Breaft and Covert-feathers of the Tail, both above and beneath, are Blue; the middle of the Belly is Black, which part is cover'd by the Wing in the Pofture it is drawn; behind the black Part of the Belly is a white Mark acrofs the Vent, the Quill-feathers, and the Row of Coverts next above them, are of a dirty purplifh Colour in both Birds, as they are in moft of this Kind; the Tails in both Birds are Black above, and Blue beneath; the Legs and Feet alfo in both are Black.

THE fecond Bird, which I believe to be the Hen of the above defcrib'd, differs from that in the Colour of the Green, on the Head, Neck, and Coverts of the Wing, which are of a much yellower Green; the Top of the Head, upper Part of the Neck and Back, being intermixed with a red Colour; it wants the white Bar acrofs the lower Belly or Vent, in all other Particulars the above Defcription will anfwer to this.

The firft Bird was lent me by *James Theobald*, Efq; the other by *Taylor White*, Efq; From what particular Part they came, I could not be informed; but we know that *America* only produces thefe Birds, and chiefly between the Tropicks, they being rarely met with far without the Tropicks, and not at all in Winter. Near the Equinoctial they continue all the Year, as I have been informed.

THIS *Fly* is Yellow, fpotted with Black; the Eyes are redifh, the Wings are tranfparent, the greater Wings a little thick toward their fetting on, and of a browner Colour, which parts are diftinguifhed by crofs Hatching between the Veins of the Wings, there are two dark Spots in the Ends of each of the larger Wings, the leffer Wings are of an equal Clearnefs without Spots.

This *Fly* came from *Amboina*, and was lent me by Mr. *Dandridge* I need not mention the Size of the Infects here figur'd, becaufe they will all be juft of the natural Size.

The

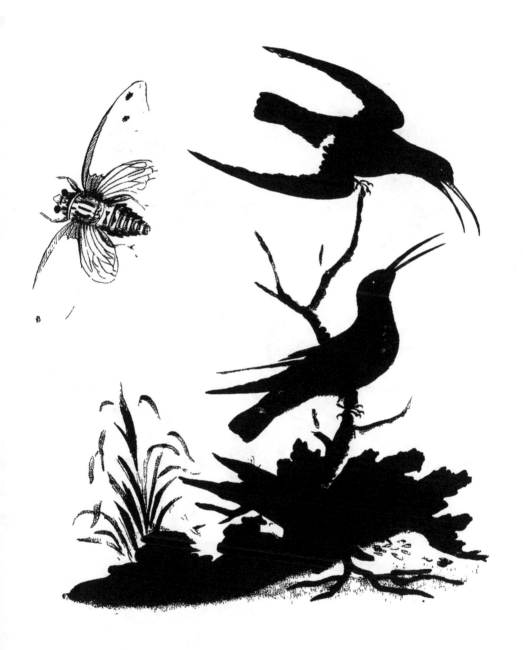

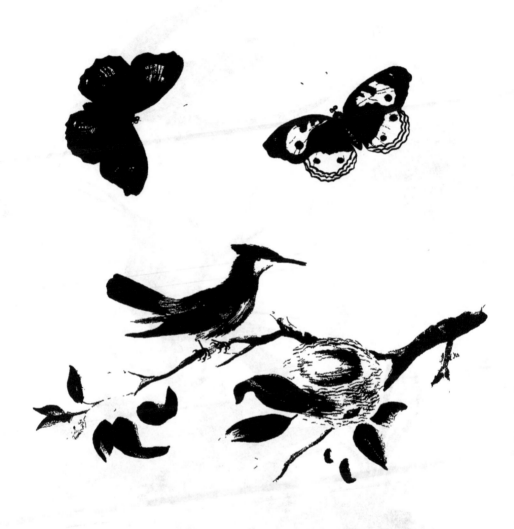

The CRESTED HUMING BIRD.

THIS Bird, with its Neft, is reprefented of its natural Bignefs; the Bill is flender, fharp-pointed, and not fo long as in moft of this Kind, of a black Colour, and very little bowed downward; the Top of the Head, from the Bill to the hinder Part, which ends in a Creft, is firft Green, and toward the hinder Part, dark Blue, both thefe Colours fhine with a Luftre far exceeding the brighteft polifh'd Metals, the green Part efpecially, which is the lighteft in fome Lights, changes from Green to Gold-colour, fo beautiful as not to be expreffed by Colours, or hardly conceiv'd in the Abfence of the Object, the Feathers of the upper Part of the Body and Wings are dark Green, intermixed with Gold-colour, juft beneath the Bill is a Spot of dirty White, the Breaft and Belly are of a dark, dirty, grifled or mixed Gray-colour, the Quills are of a Purple-colour, the Tail is of a bluifh Black, fomething glossy on the upper Side, the under Side more glossy than the upper, which is not common, the Legs and Feet are very fmall, and black of Colour. The Neft is compos'd of a very fine foft cotton or filky Subftance, I could not tell which; there is in it a Mixture of two Sorts, the one Red, the other of a yellowifh White, it is hung between two little Twigs, as exprefs'd. The young Leaves and Rudiments of the Fruit were on the Branch, which by Comparifon with the Defcription, feems to be the *Sweet Sop-tree.* Sloan's *Natural Hiftory of* Jamaica, *Vol.* 2 *Page* 168. *Tab.* 227 The Fruit, when Ripe, is of the Bignefs of a *Turkey's* Egg.

Mr. *John Warner* obliged me with a Sight of this Bird and Neft. He had it of a Captain who brought it from the *Weft Indies.*

THESE *Flies,* which I take to be Male and Female, were brought from *China,* the Bodies in both are Brown, the Wings in the firft *Fly* are border'd all round with Black, the upper Wings have each one large irregular Spot of Orange-colour, and a few fmall ones at their Extremities, the lower Wings have alfo a pretty large Spot of Orange-colour in each Wing, and near the Body a large Spot of Blue, encompafs'd with Black, which appears partly cover'd by the upper Wings, befide thefe, there are two Half-moon-like Spots, and fome dirty Marks of Orange-colour in the Black round their Borders. In the fecond *Fly,* the Wings are border'd with dirty Brown or Black, the middle Parts of both upper and under Wings are of a faint Yellow-colour, there are blue Spots furrounded with Black near the Body, in the lower Wings, in each Wing, both upper and under, are two Eyes, whofe Middles are Blue, circled round with Black, the three little tranfverfe Bars which border on the outer Part of the outer Wings are very Black, the lower Wings are border'd with two Rows of brown Scolops.

L   *The*

The RED-THROATED HUMING BIRD.

THESE Birds, which I am pretty well assured are Cock and Hen, together with the Nest and Eggs, are represented of their natural Size; the first or Cock-bird has already been very well done by Mr. *Catesby*, in his History of *Carolina*, yet I did not care to leave him out of this Plate, since I have the Hen, Nest and Eggs; the Bills are long, slender, straight, and of a black Colour in both; the upper Part of the Head, Neck, Back, and lesser Coverts of the Wings in both, are of a fine silky-looking dark Green, which seems to be intermixed with very fine golden Threads; the prime Feathers in the Wings of both are of a dirty Purple-colour, as they are in all or most *Huming Birds*, in the Cock the Tail is Purple, except the middle Feathers, which are Green, the middle of the Belly and Covert-feathers under the Tail are White, the Sides under the Wings Green, like the Back; but what chiefly distinguishes the Cock from the Hen, is a most beautiful shining Scarlet-colour under the Chin, which reaches to the Breast, changing its Colour in different Positions to the Light, sometimes into a deep Sable-colour, then again to the Colour of shining Gold, the Feathers in this red Part are firm and regularly placed, like the Scales of Fish; the Hen differs from the Cock, in that her whole under Side is white from Bill to Tail, and the Purple Feathers of her Tail are tip'd with White, the middle Feathers being Green; the Legs and Feet in both, are very small and of a black Colour; the Nest, which was fastened on the upper Side of a Branch, was compos'd of a woolly Substance and Moss, the inside being Wooll or some soft Substance, of a light yellowish brown Colour; the outside is cover'd with Moss very firmly and closely laid together, which is not easily ruffled with slight handling; the Eggs are small and white, seeming to be no sharper at one End than the other, as is common to most Eggs.

Mr. *Peter Colinson*, F. R. S. oblig'd me with a Sight of this curious Pair of Birds and Nest. They are found in *Carolina*, and as far North as *New England* in the Summer Season, but retire Southward, or disappear in Winter. I have been informed that no Bird of this Genus, except this one, ever visits the *English* Colonies in *North America*.

❦❦❦❦❦❦❦❦❦❦ ❦❦❦ ❦❦ ❦❦❦❦❦❦❦❦❦❦❦ ❦❦

THIS *Fly* is of a black or dark Sable-colour, having a pretty large scarlet Spot across each of the upper Wings, beside some Streaks of the same Colour near the Body, the lower Wings have each four little round red Spots near the Body. I know not from what Part this *Fly* came. I had it of Mr *William Goupey*.

The

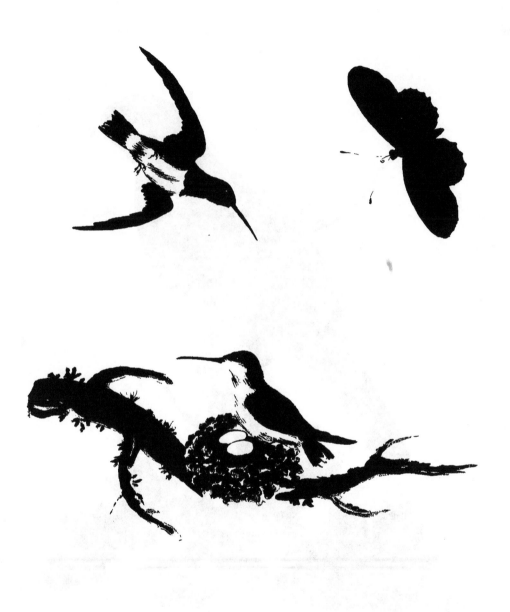

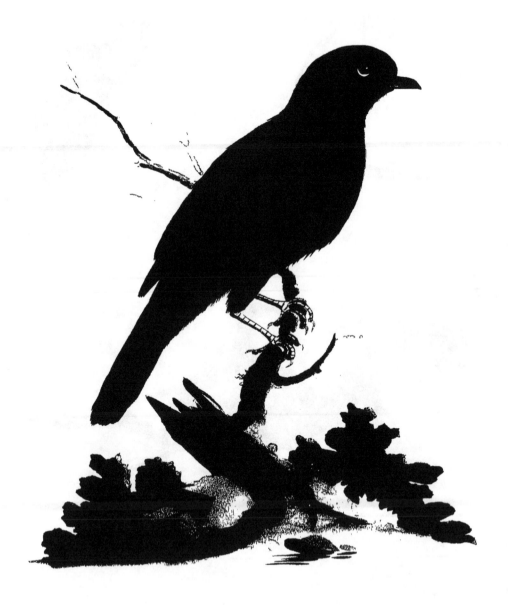

The RED BIRD *from* Surinam.

IT is of the Size here figur'd, and of the Tribe or Family of that I have defcrib'd under the Name of the *Golden-headed Black Tit-moufe*, the Feet in both agreeing with the *King-fifher's*, the Bill is of a middling Length and Thicknefs, not flender as in *Larks*, nor thick at its Bafis, as in the *Finch*-kind, the Top of it a little arched, of a dirty red Colour, the Corners of the Mouth deep cleft, the Eyes are placed juft over the Slits of the Mouth, the Top of the Head, lower Part of the Belly, Thighs, Rump, Tail and its Covert-feathers, are of a beautiful Red or Scarlet-colour, the Sides of the Head, Neck, Breaft, Back, and Wings, are of a dull dirty Red-colour, very dark all round the bright Red on the Crown, lighter on the Sides of the Head and Breaft, the Red on the hinder Part of the Neck and Back is very dark, almoft dusky, the Reds vary in Shades alfo in the Wings, the Tips of the Coverts being darkifh, and the Quills toward their Tips gradually becoming almoft Black, the Tail-feathers at their Tips are Black for about half an Inch in Breadth; the Legs, Feet, and Claws, are of a dirty yellow Colour, the hinder Part of the Legs have fmall Feathers or Hairs down to the Feet.

This Bird is in the Duke of *Richmond*'s Cabinet. By the Make of its Feet, I take it to be a Bird frequenting watery Places At firft Sight it feems not unlike the *Cardinal Crefted Red Grofs-beck*, or as we call it, the *Virginia Nightingale*, tho' it differs very much from that in the Bignefs and Shape of the Bill, which in that is *Finch*-like, and of a very large Size in Proportion; the Bill in this is rather fmall than large; this wants the Creft, tho' I believe it can raife the Feathers on the Crown, they being pretty long and loofe, that hath a manifeft Creft, which appears hanging backward when not erected, for Magnitude, they are pretty equal. I could name this Bird only from its Colour and Country, not knowing what Genus of *European* Birds to range it with. Were it not for the Structure of the Feet, this Bird might be ranged with the *Garrulus Bohemicus*, or *Silk-tail*, it being much of the fame Bignefs and Make of Body, and the Bill very like it This Bird being fomething doubtful as to its Genus, I have faid the more concerning it, that the Learned and Curious may hereafter be able to fix it more certainly

The GOWRY BIRD.

THIS Bird is of the *Groos-beck* or *Finch*-kind, of the Size here re-prefented. *Albin* has figur'd a Bird fomething like this, and makes it the Hen of another Bird he has placed it with; he calls it a *Chinefe Sparrow* in his *Hiftory of Birds, Vol. 2. Tab.* 53. I do not think it the Hen of the Bird he has figur'd with it. I have feen feveral of thefe Birds at Dr. *Monroe's,* and at other Gentlemen's Houfes, and I find they vary pretty much, as do the little *Indian* Birds call'd *Amadebats:* So that every Bird would require a feparate Defcription. The Bird here under-defcrib'd, was one of the fineft I have met with; the Bill is of the Shape and Bignefs of our *Green-Finch's* Bill, of a Lead-colour, yet the Bird exceedeth not half the Size of the *Green-Finch;* the Eyes are of a dark Hazel-colour; the Head, Neck, beginning of the Breaft, Back, Wings, and Tail, are of a dark redifh Brown; the fore Part of the Neck hath fomething of a purplifh Caft, the greater Quills are of a dirtier Brown than the reft of the Wing, the Rump is of a lighter greenifh Brown; the Breaft, quite acrofs, and the Belly on the Sides, is black, thickly fprinkled with fmall round white Spots, of the Size of Rape-feed, fome a little bigger, others a little lefs; the middle of the Belly, Thighs, lower Belly, and Covert-feathers under the Tail, are light Brown, or dirty White; the Legs and Feet are of a bluifh or Lead-colour, fhaped as in other fmall Birds.

Charles du Bois, Efq; Treafurer to the *India* Company, invited me to his Houfe to draw this Bird. He told me it came from the *Eaft Indies,* and was called a *Gowry* or *Coury Bird,* they being fold for a fmall Shell apiece, call'd a *Gowry;* fo that I believe it doth not come from *China, Gowrys* not pafling there as Money.

THE *Beetle* is of its natural Size, and all over of a bright fhining brownifh Black; it came from the *Eaft Indies,* and was given me by my good Friend Mr. *Pope,* of *Ratcliff,* a Gentleman well known for many curious and ufeful Inventions, particularly for Marbling Paper with a Margent, to prevent Frauds in the publick Offices; for the fole doing of which, his Majefty has given him Licence under his Broad Seal. I am oblig'd to this Gentleman for many curious Things.

The

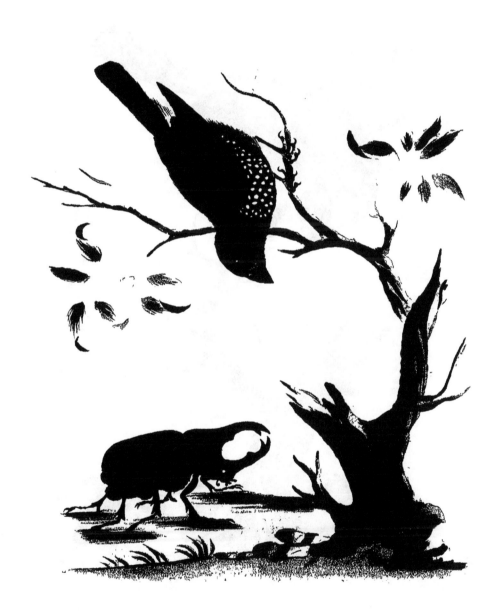

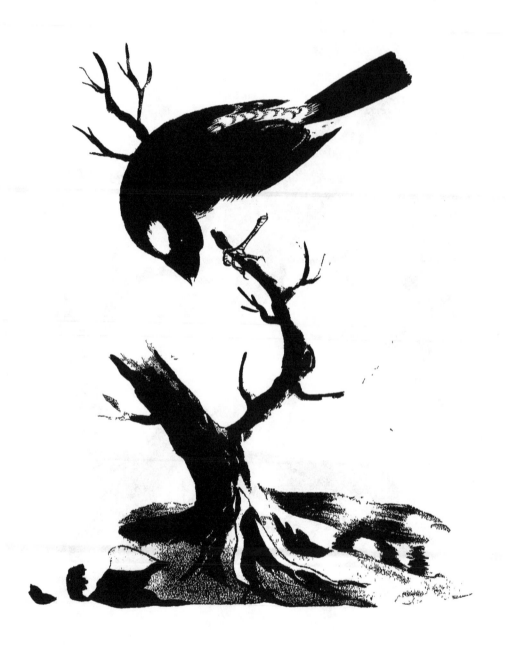

The Cock PADDA *or* RICE-BIRD.

THIS Bird is figur'd of its natural Bigness; it is about the Size of a *Green-Finch,* or rather bigger; it hath a very thick Bill for the bigness of the Bird, ending in a Point, of a fine red Colour above and beneath in the thick Part toward the Head, the Point for a little Space is White; the Eye is of a dark Colour; the Eyelids or Border of Skin round the Eye is of a bright Red; the Head is Black, except a white Spot on each Cheek, of the Shape of a Kidney-bean; the Neck, Breast, Back, and Covert-feathers of the Wings are of a fine bluish Ash-colour, the Rump of a lighter Ash-colour than the Back; the Ash-colour on the Breast changes gradually toward the Belly, into a faint Rose or Blossom-colour; beyond this Colour the lower Belly and Covert-feathers under the Tail, are dirty White; the greater Quill-feathers, and the whole Tail, are of a black Colour; the Legs and Feet of a faint Red, the Claws of a dirty White-colour. Tho' this Bird has but little gay Colouring in it, yet is it a Bird of much Beauty, the Feathers all over, except the Wings, appear to have a fine soft Bloom on them, like that on Plumbs, and fall on one another in such Order that no Feather can be distinguished, but the whole appears with a Surface smooth and even. I saw one of these Birds alive at Sir *Hans Sloane*'s: They came from *China.*

As there are Figures join'd with all these Descriptions, in which great Care has been taken justly to express the extreme Parts, such as the Bills and Feet, and other Parts which distinguish the Genus or Species of the different Birds, I thought it not proper to trouble the Reader with long and perplexed Descriptions of those Parts, since he can, by casting his Eye on the Figure, convey to his Sense a much perfecter Idea, than a laborious and just Description in Words could give.

M

The *Hen* PADDA *or* RICE-BIRD.

THIS Bird is altogether of the same Magnitude and Shape with the last describ'd, to which I suppose it to be the Hen. It is by the People who bring them from *China*, call'd the *Padda Bird*, because they are fed with that Grain ; *Padda* being the Name by which Rice is call'd, while the Grain continues in the Husks ; so that I think the *Rice Bird* not a very improper Name. They are said very much to annoy the Plantations of Rice ; but tho' I have given it this Name, yet I must take notice these Birds are of that Tribe or Family of small Birds we in *England* call *Finches*, tho' their Bills are larger in Proportion than any of that Genus we have with us. I not having Opportunity of seeing this Bird alive, the Description may be less perfect than the other. It was preserv'd in Spirits at Sir *Hans Sloane*'s.

The Bill is of a Flesh-colour, it hath also the Eyelids or Skin round the Eye of a Flesh-colour ; the Head is wholly Black, wanting the white Spots in the Cheeks, which is the principal Difference between this and the last describ'd Bird ; the Neck, Back, Breast, and Wings, are of an Ash-colour, not so bright as in the former, the Belly gradually changing into a faint dirtyish Blossom-colour, the Quills something darker than the Covert-feathers of the Wings ; on the Ridge of the Wing next the Breast, is a white Spot ; the lower Belly, and Coverts under the Tail, are White, the Tail is Black, the Legs and Feet of a Flesh-colour ; the Edges of the Feathers, as in the other, intermix so equally, as to appear more like fine Hair than Feathers.

Some People using the *India* Trade, who have seen these Birds, call them *Java Sparrows*, and others, *Indian Sparrows*, and affirm they are found in *Java* ; if so, it is like they are found in most of the Countries to which our *India* Company trade ; but I rather believe the Trade between *China* and *Java*, may have made them as Plenty as Cage-Birds in *Java*, from which some may have supposed them Natives of that Country. I have observ'd Figures of these Birds very frequently in *Chinese* Pictures, which is a pretty convincing Argument they are Natives of *China*.

The

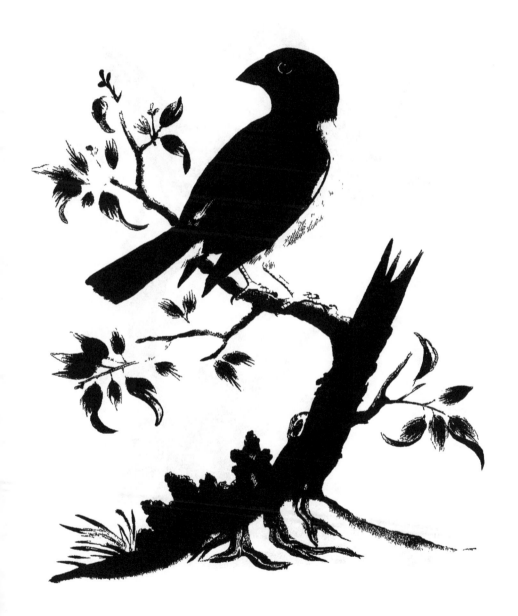

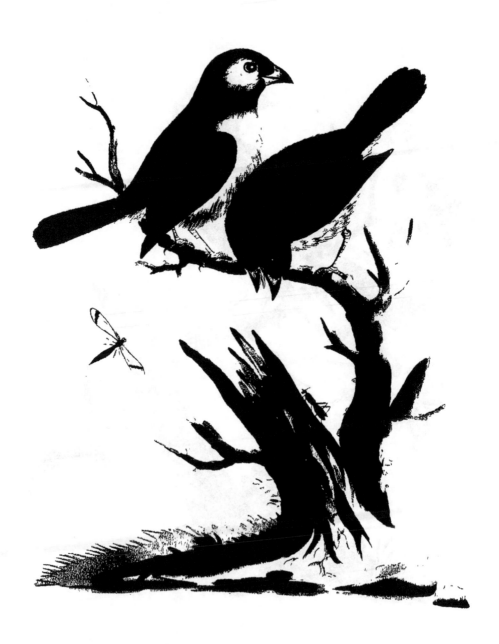

The CHINESE SPARROWS.

THESE Birds are figur'd of their Natural Bigneſs; they are of the *Finch*-kind, tho' they have Bills of a larger Size, the Bills in both are very large, juſt of the ſame Shape and Bigneſs, of a light bluiſh Aſh-colour, the Head, in the firſt Bird, which I ſuppoſe to be the Cock, is Black; in the fore Part of the Neck, the Black reaches down to the Breaſt, the Eye is of a dark-Colour; the whole Body, Wings, and Tail, are of an equal Red-brown or dark Cinnamon-colour, the Legs and Feet of an Aſh-colour.

THE ſecond Bird, which I ſuppoſe to be the Hen, hath a dark-colour'd Eye, the Sides of the Head, round the Eye, the under-ſide of the Neck, Breaſt, Belly, and Covert-feathers under the Tail, are of a dirty White, a little inclining to a faded Bloſſom-colour; the Top of the Head, hinder Part of the Neck, Back, and Wings, are of a dirty brownish Aſh-colour, the upper Covert-feathers of the Tail, White; the Tail and greater Quill-feathers, are of a Black or Dusky-colour, the Legs and Feet are of a Fleſh-colour.

I drew theſe Birds at a Bird-Merchant's in *White-Hart Yard* in the *Strand*, who call'd them *Indian Sparrows*. They were in a Cage together, and ſeem'd to agree like Cock and Hen. Though *Albin* has figur'd this with a black Head, and a Bird different to what I have here placed with it, which he ſays is the Hen; I ſhould not have repeated *Albin*'s Bird, had not this I call the Hen, been a Bird not yet deſcrib'd. *Albin*'s Cock differs from mine, in that it hath a broad black Stroke drawn from the Breaſt downward, through the whole Length of the Belly, which I could not diſcover, though I have, ſince I made this Draught, had one of theſe Birds myſelf, and examin'd it narrowly to find this Mark, but found the Belly wholly of the red Ruſſet-colour. I have been told theſe Birds are brought from *China* I have given it Mr. *Albin*'s Name, which I think not improper, beſides, a multiplicity of Names for the ſame Thing, cauſes much Confuſion in Natural Hiſtory. See *Albin*'s Figure in *Vol. 2*. *Plate* 53 of his *Hiſtory of Birds*

The YELLOW-HEADED LINNET.

THIS Bird being of Kin to *Linnets* or *Canary-Birds*, I choose to call it by this Name: I have heard them call'd *Mexican Sparrows*; but I think it more of the *Linnet*-kind; the Bill is moderately big, like the Bills of most of our hard-bill'd Birds who crack Seeds, of a whitish or pale Flesh-colour; the Eye is of a Hazel-colour; the Head and Throat are of a yellow Colour; from behind the Eyes, down the Sides of the Neck, are drawn brown Marks, growing wider towards their lower Parts, and falling into the Back; the hinder Part of the Head, upper Side of the Neck, Back, Wings, and Tail, are of a dirty Brown-colour, spotted on the Neck and Back with dirty Spots, drawn downward; the greater or outer Quills, and the Feathers of the Tail darker than the Back, and upper Part of the Wings; the Breast, Belly, Thighs, and Covert-feathers under the Tail, are of a light Clay-colour, the Breast and Belly spotted, with dark brown Spots, drawn downward, which Spots begin on the lower Part of the Yellow on the Throat; the Legs and Feet are Brown, or of a dirty Flesh-colour.

I drew this Bird at Sir *Charles Wager*'s House at *Parsons Green*. The Print shews the Bird of its natural Bigness.

A Cage of these Birds was found on board a *Spanish* Prize, taken by an *English* Ship in the *West Indies*; they are Natives of *Mexico*, the Ship in which they were found being bound from *Vera Cruz* to *Old Spain*.

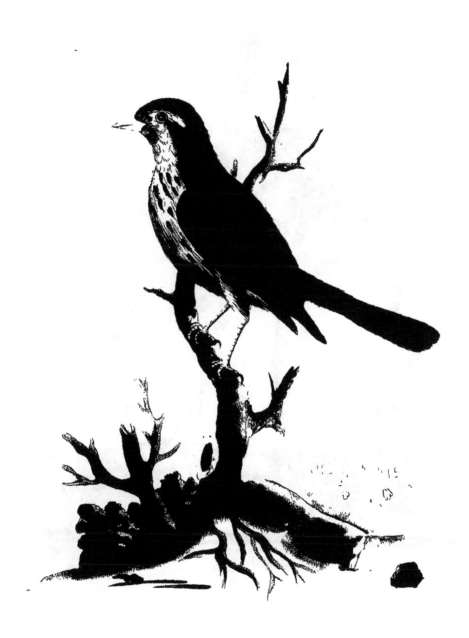

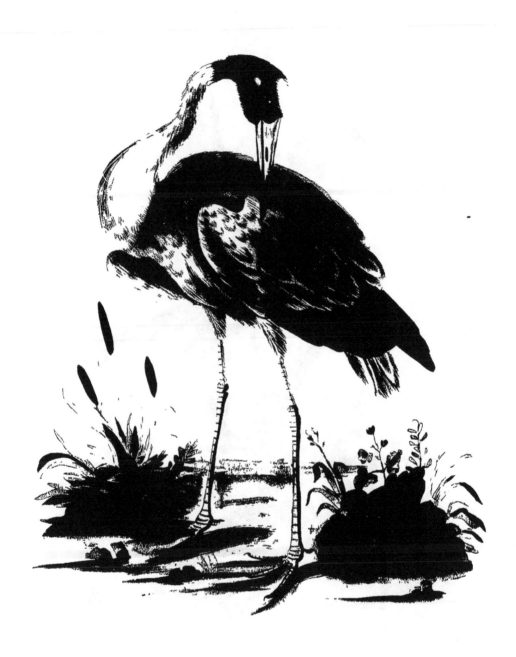

The GREATER INDIAN CRANE.

THIS is a very large and ftately Bird, I believe bigger than the common *Crane*, and hath a longer Bill in Proportion; it walks with a very grave and folemn Air; its Height, as it ftands or walks, without extending the Neck greatly, is about five Feet. Mr. *Willughby* has defcrib'd an *Indian Crane* which feems to be much lefs than this, and a quite different Bird; fo I thought the *Greater Indian Crane* might be a Name proper enough for this Bird; it fed on Barley and other Grain, but by reafon of the Length and Sharpnefs of the Bill, it could not gather the Grain into its Mouth without jerking back its Head pretty quick, and catching the Grain into its Mouth after it had taken it in the Point of its Bill; the Bill is long and pretty thick toward the Head, ending in a fharp Point, of a greenifh Yellow-colour, dusky at the Tip, having on each Side an oblong Noftril pretty near the Middle, tho' nearer the Head than the Point, the Eyes are of a bright hazel or redifh Colour; the Head, and a fmall Part of the Neck, are cover'd with a bare Skin, of a fine red Colour; about the Bafe of the Bill, under the Chin, and all round the beginning of the Neck, or hinder Part of the Head, it is thin fet with fine black hair-like Feathers, a fmall Space of the Neck remaining quite bare below it; the Crown of the Head, and two Spots by the Ears are White, and bare of Feathers; the Neck is very long, cover'd in the upper Part with white Feathers, which gradually become Afh-colour towards its Bottom; the Neck feathers are not fo long and loofe as in *Herons*, the whole Body, Wings and Tail, except the greater or outer Quills of the Wings, are Afh-colour, fomething lighter on the Breaft than on the Back and Wings, the Quills are Black, and extend themfelves, when the Wings are clofed, of almoft equal Length with the Tail, the Legs are very long and bare of Feathers for a good Space above the Knees, it hath three Toes ftanding forward, of a moderate Length, and a fmall back Toe, both Legs and Feet are of a red Colour like thofe of *Pigeons*, the Claws black.

This Bird I drew from the Life at Sir *Charles Wager*'s, who afterwards prefented it to Dr *Mead*. It was brought from the *Eaft Indies*.

N   *The*

The COOT-FOOTED TRINGA.

THIS Bird is here figur'd of the natural Bignefs; it is for Shape, Size, and general Colouring, like the *Leffer Tringa*, or the *Stint*, defcrib'd in *Willughby*, the chief Difference being in the Feet, which are border'd with fcollop'd Fins, as in the *Bald Coot*; the Bill is long, pretty flender, and of a black Colour, a little bowed downward at the Point of the upper Mandible; the Eyes are placed pretty far from the Bill, as they are in moft of this Kind; the Crown of the Head is Black; the Sides of the Head, all round the Eyes, round the Bafe of the Bill and Chin, are White; the whole Neck is of a faint Afh-colour, a very little inclining to Bloffom-colour; the Breaft, Belly, Thighs, and Covert-feathers under the Tail are White; the lower Part of the Neck behind, the whole Back, Wings, and Tail, are of a dark dirty Brown-colour, tho' the very Borders of the Feathers are fringed with a lighter Colour; the greater or outer Quills are almoft black, having white Shefts or Stems, the middle Quills have white Tips and Borders pretty narrow, the inner or thofe next the Back, of the fame Colour with it; the Covert-feathers next above the Quills, are tip'd with White pretty deep, which form a broad white Bar acrofs the Wing, the under Side of the Tail is Afh-colour; the Legs are of a middling Length, bare above the Knees for a good Space; it hath four Toes ftanding after the ufual Manner, the three forward Toes have fcollop'd Fins on each Side, according to the num-ber of Joints in each Toe, the Indentures falling in upon every Joint, fo that the Fins are not difturbed or ruffled by the bending of the Joints, the back Toe is fmall, both Legs and Feet are of a Lead-colour; it hath black Claws. I look on this Bird's Feet to be very fingular, no Bird of the *Snipe* or *Tringa*-kind having any thing like them.

It was given me by Mr. *Alexander Light*, a curious Perfon, now re-fiding in *Hudfon's Bay*, whither he was fent by the *Hudfon's Bay* Com-pany. He told me it came on board a Ship failing on the Coaft of *Maryland*, a good Diftance from Shore, in an Off-land Wind.

The

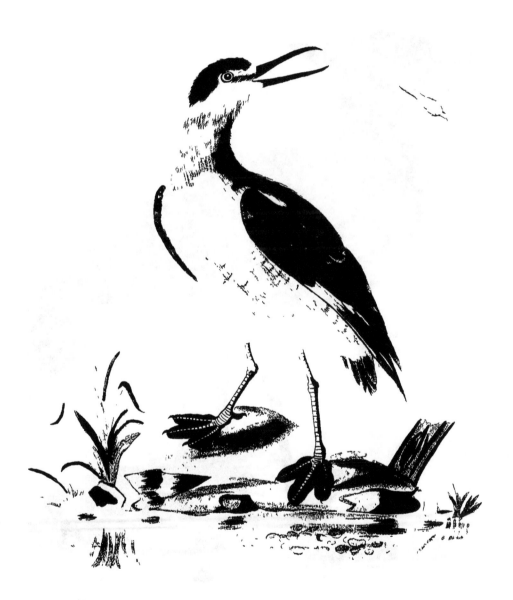

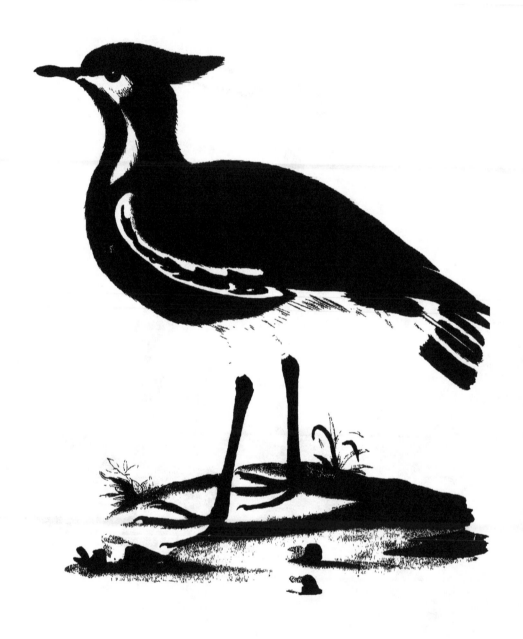

The BLACK-BREASTED INDIAN PLOVER.

THIS Bird is fomething bigger than the *Lapwing*, it agrees pretty near in Size with our *Englifh Grey* and *Green Plovers*, being fhap'd like them, except in its Legs, which are a pretty deal longer; it is here drawn of its natural Bignefs; its Bill is of a middling Length, of a pretty equal Thicknefs, black of Colour, ending in a Point, the Middle of the Bill is not quite fo thick as it is at its Bafis and near the Point; it hath on each Side an oblong Noftril; the Crown of the Head is Black with a green Glofs, thefe black Feathers reach an Inch beyond the Head behind, and form a Creft; the Cheeks, hinder Part of the Head, and two broad Lines down on each Side the Neck are White; between the black Crown and the White in the Sides of the Head, are placed the Eyes; the lower Part of the Neck behind, the whole Back and Covert-feathers of the Wings, are of a brown Colour; the Tips of the Rows of Coverts next above the Quills are White, the greater Quills Black, the leffer next the Back, Brown; the Ridge of the Wing, from the Bend downward, hath black and white Feathers intermixed; from the Bill downward, on the Throat, and beginning of the Breaft, is drawn a black Mark, which falls into the Black on the Breaft; the Breaft and part of the Belly are Black, having a fine purple Glofs on the Breaft; the Thighs, lower Belly, and Covert-feathers under the Tail are White; the Feathers of the Tail are of equal Length, White at their Bottoms, and Black acrofs the End, for the breadth of an Inch and a half; the Legs are longer than common in this kind of Birds; it hath only three Toes of a moderate Length all ftanding forward, the Legs are bare of Feathers a little way above the Knees; both Legs, Feet and Claws, are of a dirty dark Brown, inclining to Black.

I drew this from a Bird lent me by Mr. *Peter Colinfon*, which was fent in Spirits with other Birds from *Gamron* in *Perfia*. I wrote it from *Bengal* on the Plate, through a Miftake.

The SPUR-WINGED WATER HEN.

THIS Bird is of the *Water Hen*-kind, *Willughby* has defcrib'd fomething like it as to Shape, but of other Colours, the Print fhews the Bird of its natural Bignefs, the Bill is near an Inch and a half long, of a yellow Colour, the Noftrils fituate on each Side about the middle of the Bill; it hath at the Bafis of the upper Mandible a bald Skin, as in other *Water Hens*, but different, in that it is a loofe Flap, fcollop'd with three Scollops on the Top, join'd to the Head at the Bottom, of a yellowifh Colour; I fuppofe it was Red when the Bird was living, fince that Part is defcrib'd to be fo in the Birds *Margrave* faw in *Brafil*, the Crown of the Head is Brown, intermixed with fome dusky Spots, from the Corners of the Mouth, through the Eyes, to the hind Part of the Neck on each Side, is drawn a black Line, above the Eyes are white Lines; the under Side of the Head, Neck, Breaft, Belly, Thighs, and under Coverts of the Tail are White, on the Sides of the Belly and Thighs, are fprinkled a few red Marks; the hinder Part of the Neck is Black, which by degrees becomes Brown in the beginning of the Back, the lower Part of the Back, Rump, and upper Side of the Tail, are of a purplifh inclining to a red Rofe-colour, the Feathers about the Shoulders, or fetting on of the Wings, are of a light Brown, the Quills of the Wings are of a fine Green-colour tip'd with Black, except a few of the fmaller next the Back, which are Brown; the firft Coverts above the Quills are Black, next above is a Row of Brown, the reft of the Coverts are of a Rofe or purplifh Colour, the Covert-feathers within-fide the Wings, are of a redifh Brown, what is moft extraordinary in this Bird, is a Pair of ftrong, thick, fhort, yellow Spurs on the Joints of the Wings turning inward, fo that they point toward each other, the Legs are very long, and bare of Feathers above the Knees; the middle Toe for Length, equals the Leg, the fide Toes a little fhorter, the back Toe is pretty long, having a Claw or Nail ftraight like a Needle, and longer than the Toe, which together equal the Length of the Leg, the back Toe is only one Joint, the inner two, the middle three, and the outer Toe four. I have been the more particular in defcribing the Joints of the Toes in this Bird, becaufe this Kind is faid in the Defcriptions I find in *Willughby* to have four Joints in each Toe, the three forward Toes have long flender Claws, pretty ftraight, both Legs, Feet and Claws of a Lead or bluifh Afh-colour.

This Bird had been preferv'd a good while in Spirits by Sir *Hans Sloane*, who lent it me that I might make a Drawing of it. I was told it was brought from *Carthagena* in *South America*.

The

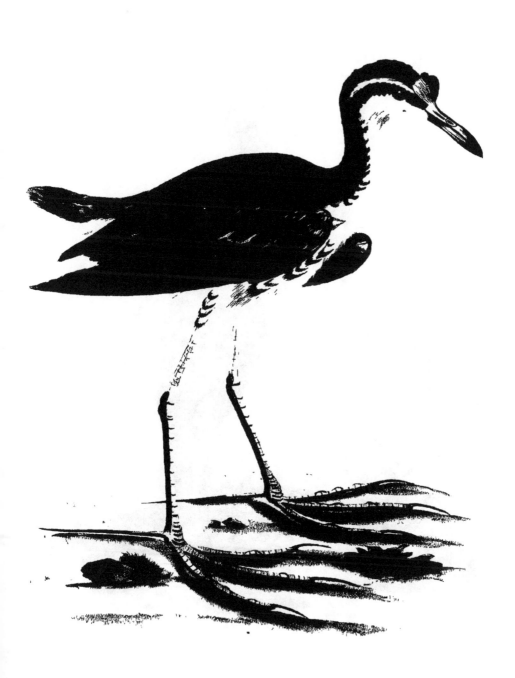

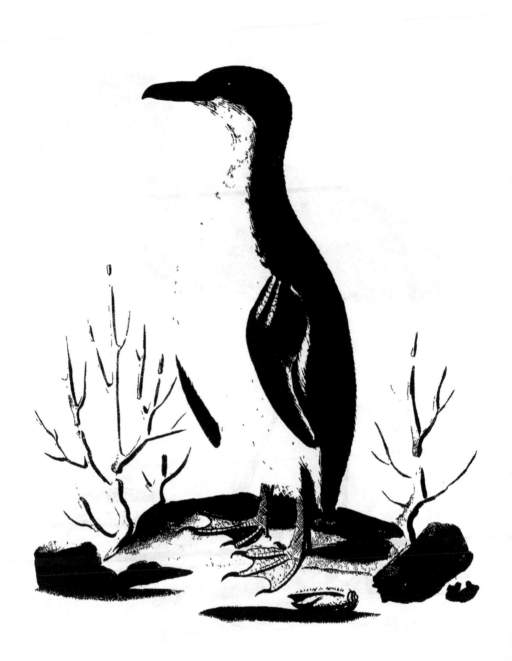

The PENGUIN.

THIS Bird is about the Bigness of a common tame *Goose*, and is suppos'd when it cometh to Land to walk in this erect Posture, by reason of the backward Situation of the Legs. Voyagers who have seen this Bird, report it to walk erect, the Bill is not very long nor depress'd like a *Goose*'s, but rather compress'd side-ways, the Corners of the Mouth are pretty deep and reach almost under the Eyes, in the upper Mandible on each Side, is a Cleft or Groove, the Feathers of the Head pointing on each Side of the Bill, and cover the Nostrils, the Bill is of a red Colour, the fore part of the Head, all round the Bill, and as far as the Eyes, is of a dirty Brown, the back Part of the Head, upper Part of the Neck and Back are of a dark dirty purplish Colour, cover'd with very small stiff Feathers, not easily ruffled or disorder'd, appearing more like the Scales of Serpents than Feathers; the under Side of the Neck, Breast, Belly, and Sides under the Wings are white, compos'd of Feathers more agreeing with the common Make and Appearance of Feathers, yet lying pretty close and firm, the Wings are small and flat, like little Boards or Paddles, of a brown Colour, both above and beneath, they are cover'd with Feathers so stiff and small, that a slight Observer might take them for Shagreen, that Part which answers the Tips of the Quills in other Wings, is white, it hath no appearance of a Tail, except a few short black Bristles on the Rump, the Legs are short, it hath three Toes standing forward, and webed together as in Geese, the inner of these Toes having a Fin or lateral Membrane within-side, a very small fourth Toe loose from the other three, standing forward and within the innermost of the other three, contrary to any thing in the Feet of Birds I have yet seen; the Legs and Feet are of a dirty red Colour, armed with pretty long sharp brown Claws, the hind Part of the Legs and Bottoms of the Feet, are Black.

This Bird was lent me by Mr. *Peter Colinson*, he could not tell from whence it came I find them mention'd chiefly by Voyagers to the Straights of *Magellan*, and the *Cape of Good Hope*.

In Sir *Tho. R.'s Voyage to India*, I find this Account "On the Isle of *Penguin* " is a sort of Fowl of that Name, that goes upright, his Wings without Feathers, " hanging down like Sleeves, faced with White, they do not fly, but only walk in " Parcels, keeping regularly their own Quarters" Churchill's *Collect. of Voyages, Vol.* 1. *p* 767

The above-mention'd *Penguin* Isle is near the *Cape of Good Hope*. I have examin'd some of the Voyages to the Straights of *Magellan*, and find very little Account of the *Penguins* there, more than that they go upright, and burrow under the Shores So that I cannot determine the above-describ'd to be a Native of any certain Part of the World Had these Voyagers given slight Descriptions of the Things they mention, we might from thence probably have fixed its native Place

The

The SPOTTED GREENLAND DOVE.

THIS Bird is here figur'd of its natural Bigness, by comparing it with the *Green-land Dove* of *Willughby*, I find it agrees exactly in Shape and Size with that, the Bill and Legs being the very fame as to Make, tho' different in Colour, therefore I believe it to be a young Bird, before it has molted its first Feathers, the old ones being Black, except a large white Spot in each Wing, and the Legs and Feet of a fine Red. The flying Bird, in this Plate, shews the *Black Greenland Dove*, at a Distance, by way of comparing it with this, the Bill is pretty long, of a dark or black Colour, a little bowed or hooked toward the Point, the whole under-side, from Bill to Tail, is white, having very faint transverse Bars of Ash-colour; the Top of the Head, upper Side of the Neck, Back and Tail, are of a dusky Black, with transverse Bars of a deep Black, the Quills are wholly Black, the Coverts above them tip'd with White, then succeeds a Row of Black, the lesser Coverts form a large Spot of White in the upper Part of the Wing, sprinkled with Black, the Ridge and upper Part of the Wing is border'd round with Black, the Legs and Feet are of a dirty Flesh-colour, it hath three Toes only, all standing forward, armed with small Claws and webed together, it hath also Fins bordering on the insides of the inner Toes. *Albin* has figur'd a Bird in his Second *Vol. p.* 73. which he calls the Cock *Greenland Dove*, and another in *Vol* 1 *p.* 81. which he calls the Hen, I believe he may have met with something like this Hen, there being such a sort of Bird, but not the Hen of the *Greenland Dove*. Now I suppose he wanting a Cock to his Hen, and seeing in *Willughby* the Colours were few and simple, thought he might easily make it out without seeing the Bird, so he made a Plate for the Cock, which is only the direct reverse of his Hen, and has colour'd it by *Willoughby's* Description, and having never seen the Cock, he supposed it to have a Bill like that he calls the Hen; whereas the *Greenland Dove* is a bigger Bird, and hath a pretty long slender Bill, more than double the Length of his in Proportion. I thought it not amiss to rectify this Mistake in Mr. *Albin's* Works.

I had this Bird of Sir *Hans Sloane*, who kept it some time alive It was presented to him by Captain *Craycott*, who brought it directly from *Greenland*.

If it be true, that this Bird changes White in Winter, as *Willughby's* Description mentions, this might perhaps be taken in the Time it was changing from Black to White, or from White to Black. See this Bird in *Willughby*, *P.* 326. *Tab* 78. tho' to me there seems no good Proof of its changing from one Colour to another.

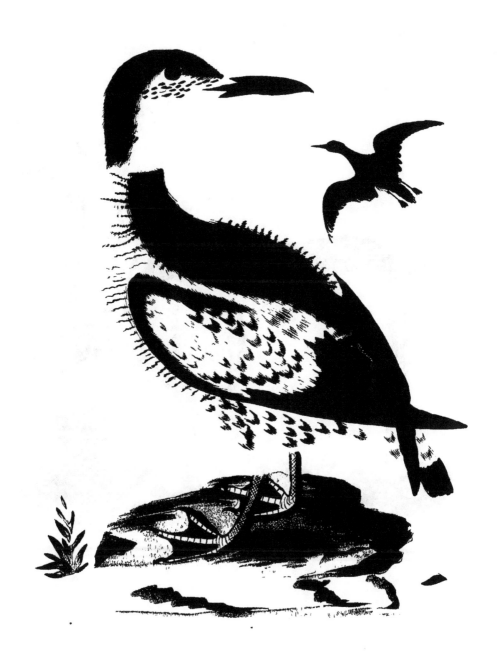

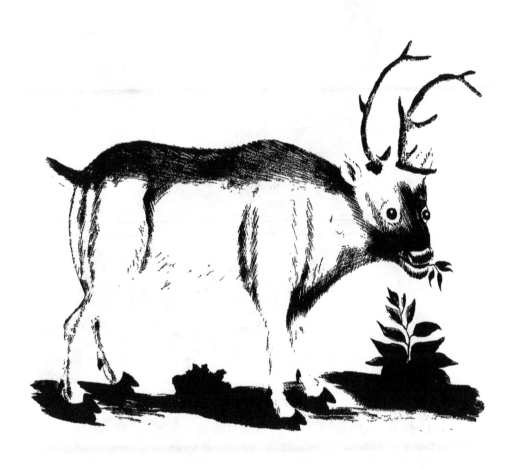

The GREENLAND BUCK.

THIS Deer, in comparison with ours in *England*, is very thick and clumsy, being for Proportion of its Parts more like a well grown Calf than a Deer; from the Ground to the top of the Shoulders, it is about three Feet high *English* measure; it hath a much shorter Neck, and thicker Legs than is common in the Deer-kind; in Summer-time it is cover'd with smooth short Hair of a Mouse-colour, against Winter there springs from beneath this a second Coat of long rough white Hair, tho' it is a little Brown on the Back, and the lower Part of the Face; this long Hair gives it a thick clumsey Appearance; in the Spring again this rough winter Clothing is, as it were, thrust off by the succeeding Summer's Coat, which is smooth and short, and so it continues to change its Coverings; what is most remarkable in this Kind is the Nose, which is wholly cover'd with Hair in that Part, which in other Deer is bare Skin and moist: I suppose had it been naked, it must necessarily have froze in those cold Countries, so Nature has given it this Covering to defend it; the Eyes are pretty large, standing a little out of the Head; both Male and Female have Horns which is not common; its Hoofs are not pointed, they part pretty much in the Cleft, and are broad at the Bottom, in order, I suppose, to keep them from sinking too far into the Snow; it hath two small Hoofs or Claws behind the greater on each Foot, placed pretty high; the Hoofs are of a dark Horn-colour; the Horns in this were not perfect, it being young; they were cover'd with a Plush-like Skin, of a brown Colour, and shap'd as in the Figure.

I saw a Head of perfect Horns brought over with these Deer, which had two large palmed Branches over the Eyes, conveniently placed as Shovels, to remove the Snow from the Grass, a little above these were two other Palms, but less, standing outward, above these each Horn spread itself into five round Branches not at all palmed. A Male and Female of these Deer were presented to Sir *Hans Sloane*, *Anno* 1738, by Captain *Craycott*, who brought them over. Sir *Hans* afterwards presented them to his Grace the Duke of *Richmond*, who sent them to his Park in *Sussex*. I hear they are since dead, without any Increase. This is by some supposed to be the Rain-Deer of the *Laplanders* and *Russians*; but I cannot pretend to assert it is, or is not. The Figure shews it in its winter Clothing.

The

The PORCUPINE *from* Hudſon's Bay.

FOR Shape and Bigneſs it much reſembles a Caſtor or Beaver, or to compare it to
ſome well known thing for Size of Body, it is equal to a Fox, tho' unlike it in
Shape, the Head is like a Rabit's; it hath a flat Noſe intirely cover'd with ſhort Hair,
the Teeth before, two above and two beneath, are very ſtrong, of a yellow Colour, and
ſeem to be made for gnawing or biting of Graſs; it hath very ſmall Ears hardly appearing beyond the Fur, the Legs are ſhort, the Claws long, four on each Foot for-
wards, and five on each hinder Foot, all hollowed within like Scoops, the Tail is of a
middling Length, thicker toward the Body than at the End, the under-ſide of the Tail
towards the End is White, it is clothed all over the Body with pretty ſoft Fur about
four Inches long, tho' ſhorter about the Head and near the Paws, and a little longer on
the hinder Part of the Head, beneath the Hair on the upper Part of the Head, Body
and Tail, it is thick ſet with very ſharp ſtiff Quills, the longeſt being hardly three Inches
long, which gradually ſhortens towards the Noſe, and on the Sides towards the Belly,
the Quills cannot be ſeen through the Fur, except a little on the Rump where the Hair
was thin; it had beſides the ſoft Fur which was all the Body over of a dark Brown or
Sable-colour, ſome long ſtiff ſtraggling Hairs thinly ſet, three Inches longer than the
under Fur, the Ends of which being of a dirty White, made the Fur appear a little
griſled in ſome Places, the Quills are very ſharp, ſeveral of them having ſtuck faſter in
my Fingers than in the Skin on a ſlight touch, they are bearded, and not eaſily drawn
out when enter'd the Skin   There came over with this, a young one about the Bigneſs
of a Rat, it had a blacker Fur than the old one, and the Quills were plainly ſeen and
felt among the Hair.

Theſe were brought from *Hudſon's Bay*, and preſented to Dr *R. M Maſſey*, and are
now in Sir *Hans Sloane*s Collection at *Chelſea*   I believe this Creature has not before
been deſcrib'd   The Quills are white with black Points   See in the Plate a Quill of
its natural Shape and Size, and the Point of a Quill magnified.

A Friend of mine reſiding at *Hudſon's Bay*, at my Requeſt has reſolved me ſome
Queries I ſent him relating to this Creature.

Extract from his Letter, dated Albany, Auguſt 10, 1742

" THE Porcupine in this Country, is a Beaſt which makes its Neſt or Den under
" the Roots of great Trees, and ſleeps much, it feeds on the Bark of Juniper
" and other Trees, but chiefly on Juniper, in Winter it eats Snow inſtead of drinking,
" and laps Water in Summer like a Cat or Dog, but carefully avoids going into it
" His Hair and Quills remain all Summer without alteration of Colour, but as the
" Weather grows warmer in the Spring, the Fur grows thinner, as in all Creatures in
" this Country.   But you may depend on better Information next Year, for they are
" very plentiful on the Eaſt Main, ſeveral of my trading *Indians* depending on them
" for Food at ſome Seaſons of the Year.

Your moſt humble Servant,
ALEXANDER LIGHT.

A

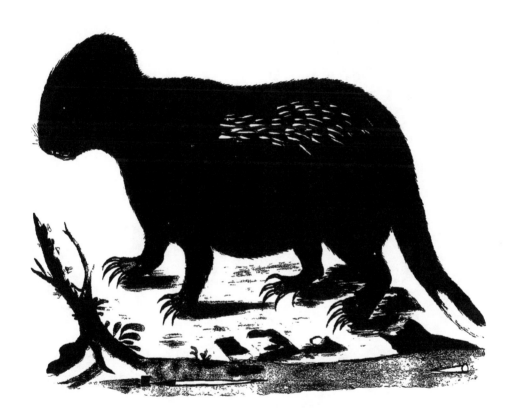